SKINNY CHICKS EAT REAL FOOD

SKINNY CHICKS EAT REAL FOOD

KICK YOUR FAKE FOOD HABIT, KICKSTART YOUR WEIGHT LOSS

CHRISTINE AVANTI, CN

WITH BONNIE BAUMAN

FOOD PHOTOGRAPHY BY NEIL HAZLE

RODALE.

© 2012 by Christine Avanti

Food photography © 2012 by Neil Hazle

Rodale books may be purchased for business or promotional use or for special sales. For information, please write to: Special Markets Department, Rodale Inc., 733 Third Avenue, New York, NY 10017

Printed in the United States of America
Rodale Inc. makes every effort to use acid-free ♾, recycled paper ♻.

Book design by Kara Plikaitis

Library of Congress Cataloging-in-Publication Data is on file with the publisher.

ISBN-13 978–1–60961–308–2

Distributed to the trade by Macmillan

2 4 6 8 10 9 7 5 3 1 hardcover

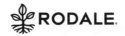

We inspire and enable people to improve their lives and the world around them.
www.rodalebooks.com

For my grandparents, Luigi and Rosemary Avanti.
Thank you for teaching me to love and respect real food.
Our family food traditions and recipes
had a tremendous influence on this book.

Contents

I Rediscover Butter

Like many in the field of nutrition, I've struggled with food issues. Having overcome my own weight-loss difficulties, I arrived at a point in my life where I watched what I ate and steered clear of fatty foods and foods high in processed carbs. So I was admittedly nervous when, in order to pursue my lifelong passion for cooking, I enrolled in culinary school. I knew that, as a student learning to cook traditional French cuisine, I'd be expected to eat all of the butter-laden foods I'd so carefully avoided for so many years.

Much to my surprise, after 9 months of cooking and eating foods like blinis with sour cream and caviar and buttery French pastries galore, I didn't gain an ounce! Plus, used to dealing with my clients' food fears in my nutritional counseling practice, I was delighted that in culinary school, not a single food was vilified—protein, unrefined carbs, and fat were all on the menu. Nothing was off the table as long as it was fresh, natural, and not processed in an unhealthy way. Not to mention the fact that, despite being exposed to so much delicious food, I wasn't driven to overeat. In fact, I began to experience a vitality and energy I hadn't had before. Best of all, I was reintroduced to a style of eating I had, without realizing it, forsaken many years earlier—*food made from fresh, whole, natural unprocessed ingredients*—"real food."

I use the word "reintroduced" because, having grown up on my grandparents' ranch, I was actually raised on a real-food diet, unlike many in the U.S. Their ranch was in Gilroy, California. My grandfather was an immigrant from Bari, Italy, and food played a central role in our family. Growing, preparing, and even preserving food was a normal part of my everyday life from the day I was born until I turned 18. My grandparents raised pigs, lambs, goats, cows, and chickens. I recall countless times helping my grandfather slice meat with an enormous meat slicer in one of our many barns. I also recall picking oranges, apples, plums, cherries, figs, persimmons, apricots, raspberries, boysenberries, prickly pears, cucumbers, green beans, squash, watermelon, artichokes, and grapes from our huge grapevines. We pickled, jarred, fermented, and prepared everything we grew, and it always tasted fabulous! So my experience cooking and eating real, natural ingredients in culinary school was like attending a reunion with old friends—friends I had ditched in favor of a low-fat, low-calorie diet after becoming immersed in the fitness culture of Los Angeles as a model and aerobics instructor in my twenties.

As it happened, I was becoming reacquainted with fresh, natural, whole ingredients about the same time a slow but steady real-food movement was taking hold. Caught up in the wave of it, I began conducting extensive research, reading the work of real-food gurus like Michael Pollan, Nina Planck, Weston Price, Marion Nestle, Mark Bittman, Sally Fallon and Mary Enig. I learned everything I could about the real-food movement. That's when I came to understand that the reason my clients (not to mention nearly the entire country) were controlled by food was that the factory food industry was actually cooking up food in its labs that was *engineered* to make consumers overeat.

And why not? The more we eat, the richer the industry grows. I learned that the highly processed foods on the American menu are designed to contain so much refined carbs, added sugar, fat, and salt, and so little fiber and nutrients, that they result in actually making us crave more fatty, salty, sugary food. This realization gave me a deeper understanding of the challenges my clients face—not to mention my own weight-loss struggles. When I was 29, my grandfather, who was really more like a father to me, passed away, and I became immersed in grief. Like so many do, I turned to food to numb my sadness. For several years, I was addicted to sweets, and I had the 30 extra pounds and the double chin to prove it. The more research I did, and the more I learned, the more convinced I became that the sugar, fat, refined carbs, and salt in factory foods were at the heart of the current obesity problem in the U.S. and in other countries that consume a Western diet. And that's when I decided to revamp my own diet program to address this problem.

Prior to this life-changing epiphany, I hadn't thought twice about recommending foods like protein bars, diet sodas, sugar substitutes, and fat-free cheese to my weight-loss clients. That's because my focus wasn't on whether the food had any added sugar or harmful additives or preservatives, or how it was processed; my focus was on whether the food would help my clients drop pounds. The first step for me toward embracing a real-food diet philosophy came when I began to understand the importance of eating to stabilize blood sugar and thus prevent cravings. In fact, this is the focus of my first book, *Skinny Chicks Don't Eat Salads*. When I began to fully embrace a real-food lifestyle, I came to understand that eating real food is the most painless way to keep blood sugar stable and avoid the cravings that come with overly processed factory foods.

My belief that the addictive qualities of factory food are behind the obesity crisis in the U.S. was cemented after I became the nutrition director and executive chef for Passages Malibu, an alcohol and drug treatment center. During my time at Passages, I came face to face with addiction. The patients at Passages were addicted to a variety of substances, including alcohol, cocaine, and heroin. However, many of the issues these folks faced with their substances of choice were the same ones my weight-loss clients face—the same cravings, feelings of powerlessness, and depression. My work at Passages also validated the weight-loss benefits of switching to a real-food diet. When I started at Passages, I gave the kitchen a complete overhaul. Refined sugars, refined flours, and any other refined carb, as well as all overly processed foods devoid of nutrition, went into the trash. In fact, many of the recipes in this book are served at Passages every week. As a result, overweight patients who enter Passages are now actually losing weight as an added bonus to their recovery. The healthy nutrition program I've instituted at Passages now plays a role in the healing process of its patients. I've gotten many letters and e-mails from patients at Passages thanking me for helping them learn to take better care of their bodies through healthy eating.

My years of helping clients with weight loss, my reintroduction to real food in culinary school, and my experience helping folks with addiction gain control of their health and weight culminated in making me realize the importance of switching to a real-food diet. For me personally, making the switch to real food from my previous factory food-laden diet was an interesting, and gradual, process. I accomplished it in stages, tackling one food issue at a time. I began by educating myself about which fats were processed in ways that did not make them dangerous or unhealthy. Then it was on to learning the dangers of refined carbs. Next, I learned about dairy and meat products. Then I turned to figuring out the whole seafood conundrum. One week I tackled salt; who knew that table salt is processed with harmful chemicals, and that 80 percent of our salt intake in this country comes from factory foods? It was a great day when I bought my first shaker of Celtic Sea Salt! Then I began hanging around farmers' markets, chatting up farmers and vendors in an effort to learn more about how they grow and raise the foods they sell.

Next, I started working with my clients to help them make the switch. I worked hard to make it easy for them to adopt a real-food diet. For example, I put together a series of "no-cook" real-food meal plans to show my clients that cooking and eating real food doesn't have to be a major production. It was important for me to prove to them that, with the right guidance, switching to a real-food diet can be done! Most importantly, I figured out the winning formula that applied real-food diets to the challenge of weight loss. That's how *Skinny Chicks Eat Real Food* was hatched.

So how does eating real food lead to weight loss? In a nutshell, consuming real food leads to weight loss as a result of the nutrients that are added to the diet—namely fiber and omega-3 fats—and the ingredients that are removed—namely added sugar, refined carbs, refined salt, and other harmful additives and preservatives that both contribute to weight gain and stand in the way of weight loss. Applying the proper balance to the diet by eating the right mix of foods at regular times guarantees weight loss. In Chapter 6 (page 57), I discuss how to achieve this balance.

The Real-Food Diet

I was inspired to write *Skinny Chicks Eat Real Food* after developing a real-food weight-loss strategy for my weight-loss clients, and I firmly believe that this is the easiest and healthiest way to shed pounds and keep them off for life. However, having made the switch from fake factory food to real food myself, I know firsthand that it's not something you do overnight. It's a three-part process. The first step is to become educated and informed about what is, and what isn't, real food. The second involves coming to terms with your current eating habits and learning how the typical American factory food diet is detrimental to both your waistline and your overall health. The final step is learning how to shop for, cook, and eat real food in the factory food world we live in. Because you have to make the switch before you can apply my weight-loss strategy, *Skinny Chicks Eat Real Food* has two jobs: First, it's a step-by-step guide through the process of making the switch from a factory food diet to a real-food diet; and second, it's a breakdown of my real-food weight-loss strategy.

Here's what you're in for in *Skinny Chicks Eat Real Food*. I believe strongly that it's vital to understand what's going on with our American factory food diet in order to grasp why it's the wrong way to nourish ourselves. Therefore, the first part of the book explains how and why the American diet is behind our nation's weight and health problems. But I've refrained from mind-numbing scientific-ese, instead serving the info straight up in plain English! Plus, I've worked hard to cut through the emotion, the confusion, and the various biases in order to get to the bottom of every issue in this section.

Chapter 1, Factory Food Is One Hell of a Drug (page 3), explores exciting new research that explains the addictive nature of overly processed food. Americans are overweight because we eat too much. We eat too much because factory food is engineered to override the biological cues that make us to stop eating when we're full. We'll take a look inside the human brain to see exactly how the sugar, other refined carbs, fat, and salt in factory food messes with your neurochemistry and causes you to overeat.

The remainder of Part I takes a shockingly candid look behind the curtain of the food industry to show you exactly how factory food gets from industrialized farm to processing plant to supermarket shelves. And because sugar and fat are two of the most prominent—and trouble-making—ingredients in the American diet, and due to the immense amount of confusion and misinformation swirling around both, each has an entire chapter devoted to it. In Chapter 3, Sugar's Bitter Side, you'll find out what's wrong with sugar and where it fits into a real-food diet. In Chapter 4, The Skinny on Fat, you'll read about what kind of fat is good for you, and what kind is bad for you, and how much of the good fat can be bad. I guarantee you'll be surprised at what you discover.

"When you know better, you do better." This is a quotation from poet Maya Angelou, and it's something I firmly believe. After reading Part I, you *will* know better, so the next part of the book is designed to allow you to take the first step toward doing better. Part II, Real-Food Recovery, begins with an explanation of which foods are "real food." It then lays out the nuts and bolts of my real-food weight-loss strategy. Chapter 7, Real Food Rehab, acknowledges that for some folks there will be a period after they stop eating addictive factory foods when they will struggle with both physical and emotional cravings. For that reason, this chapter provides readers with a big ol' box of tools they can use to get over that hump. These tools are culled from the research of the top food addiction scientists in the country as well as from real foodies who have themselves made the transition from factory food to a real-food lifestyle.

Part II forces you to face what you're really consuming when you eat a factory food diet. Research shows that people lie about what they eat—especially to themselves. Chapter 8, Reality Bites, Or What Are You *Really* Eating?, asks you to be honest with yourself about what you're eating, then gives a reality check by providing the complete lowdown on all those mysterious, impossible-to-pronounce additives that go into factory food. For instance, the innocent-sounding caramel coloring found in many soft drinks is believed to be a carcinogen, while the scarier-sounding sorbic acid and galactomannan are as natural and benign as can be. Sorbic acid, which is added to foods such as wine to prevent the growth of mold, is found in many plants, and galactomannan, often used as a thickening agent, comes from a bean. On the other hand, caramel coloring occurs when corn sugar reacts with ammonia and sulfites under high pressure at high temperatures.

Part III, Real Food in the Real World, is a comprehensive guide to putting a real-food diet into action within the reality of our dominant food system. It empowers you to make the changes needed to switch to real food, either specifically for weight loss or generally for optimal health. Among other things, Part III shows you how to navigate the factory food-filled supermarket and where to get real food outside the supermarket. And, for those looking to lose weight, Chapter 11 Real-Food Weight Loss in Action is devoted to putting the diet laid out in Chapter 6 into effect in the real world.

In addition, Part III shows you the importance of becoming a card-carrying member of a real-food community by introducing you to real-foodies in the blogosphere as well as mapping out some of the best real-food resources in the U.S. It will also turn you into a label detective so you won't fall for the factory food industry's misleading labeling and marketing ploys. Plus, you'll learn how to stock a real-food pantry, get to the bottom of what "certified organic" means, discover why sea salt is better for you than refined salt, learn how to buy "in season," and safely shop for seafood (toxins like mercury and PCBs are an unfortunate reality). And you'll get the down-low on the "raw milk" controversy. Best of all, I provide some easy-to-follow meal plans and several delicious, satisfying, real-food recipes that follow the tenets of my real-food weight-loss strategy.

Whether you're signing up for this journey to lose weight or to get real about what you eat, after you read this book you'll be forever changed. For too long we've had our health on autopilot and have allowed folks that aren't looking out for our best interests to feed us. As a result, our nation's health is spinning out of control. For the first time ever, a generation of our country's children will have a shorter lifespan than the generation that came before. It's time to take back control of what we eat. Aren't you ready to get in the driver's seat when it comes to your health and well-being and that of your family? So get ready, get set, and get real!

PART I

Addicted to Factory Food

CHAPTER 1

Factory Food Is One Hell of a Drug

When I was in my twenties, my best girlfriends and I nicknamed one of our favorite junk foods "cocaine munchies"—those mini powdered donuts that come about two dozen to a bag. Obviously, we called them "cocaine munchies" because of the powdered sugar's resemblance to that other white, powdery substance. But the donuts had something else in common with their namesake: They were downright addictive! It was impossible to eat just one. Once the bag was opened, the bag was emptied. While we were licking the powdered sugar remnants of one of them off our lips, our hands were already in the bag reaching for the next one. Back then, when we gushed that we were *"totally addicted!"* to these sweet little treats, we were unaware that our dramatics were backed by science. Fast-forward to today, and it isn't at all a stretch to say, "I'm addicted" . . . to donuts, chocolate, French fries, ice cream—heck, just insert any sweet/fatty/salty food. As I have learned working at the Passages alcohol and drug rehab facility in Malibu, California, it turns out there's a strong similarity between the pull of drugs and alcohol and the power of certain foods over our bodies and minds—a power like the one that resulted in all those powdered donuts I ate packing an extra 30 pounds on me shortly thereafter.

In this chapter, we'll take a close look at how the ingredients in certain factory foods get you hooked. Then we'll explore how those addictive foods reel us in and make us fat. Lastly, we'll take a look at the most common addictive eating traps, and I'll help you figure out which ones you've fallen into.

This Is Your Brain on a Chocolate Chip Cookie

Scientists have discovered that the same biological processes that cause us to become addicted to drugs and alcohol can cause us to exhibit addictive behavior toward food. But not just any food—no one is walking around jonesing for broccoli or obsessing about their next hit of grilled tuna topped with peach salsa. The foods under the microscope are those that contain a combination of fat and refined carbohydrates. (For the most part, the body reacts to refined white flour the same way it does to refined white sugar.) Salt plays a supporting role to the seductive combo. Foods containing particular combinations of these ingredients cause a very specific chemical reaction in our brains that is responsible for getting us hooked.

Here's a look at this reaction. Picture it: You've baked an entire batch of chocolate chip cookies. (Chocolate chip cookies are basically nothing but fat, sugar, and refined flour with a bit of salt in the mix.) You reach for a cookie, take a bite, and begin to chew. Now we're going to zero in on what's happening in your brain: While you chew that warm, fresh-out-of-the-oven cookie with its melted semi-sweet chocolate chips and its heavenly combination of vanilla and butter, what the white coats call your *opioid circuitry*—your body's primary pleasure center—becomes stimulated and releases chemicals called *opioids*. Opioids are the brain chemicals that give us that pleasurable "ooh, ahhh, mmm" feeling. In fact, the feel-good effects of opioids are similar to those of drugs like morphine.

So now you're chewing away on your second bite. By now your taste buds are completely enraptured by the combination of warm, melted chocolate tucked inside the moist and buttery cookie. Your opioid circuitry is all abuzz in your brain. Here's where things start to get a little complicated. As you're chewing, another brain system becomes stimulated: your *dopamine circuitry*, which functions as your reward center. While your opioid circuits give you the feeling of "I like," your dopamine circuits give you the feeling of "I want." Dopamine has the ability to steer our attention to a certain thing. It's what gives us the motivation to want something enough to get off the couch and pursue it.

Dopamine gives rewarding foods—like that chocolate chip cookie—center stage in our brains. The more rewarding the food, the more attention we pay it, and the more vigorously we pursue it. And get this: Our reward system happens to be one of the best performing, most finely tuned systems in the human body. When it's activated, it takes an awful lot to derail us from our goal of acquiring whatever it is we "want." Say you've made up your mind to take a ride to your favorite ice cream parlor to get a couple scoops of Ben & Jerry's Chocolate Therapy ice cream. You won't be deterred by a phone call from your mom, a traffic jam on the road, or the line at the store. On the other hand, say you've set aside time to work on your taxes. I'm betting there are easily at least 357,000 things that could cause you to postpone that plan for another day.

Okay, back to you and your batch of cookies. After you've eaten a couple of cookies, you put them away in a canister and prepare to go about your business. Maybe you have a job presentation to work on or you're just planning to do some gardening. You're trying to focus on the task at hand, but you just can't get those dang cookies out of your mind! It's getting super frustrating. A conversation begins in your head, "No, I've already had two cookies, I don't need any more!" you say to yourself. "I'm not even hungry. But they're awful good!" you reply with a sigh. Then you begin to get flashes of how it tasted and felt in your mouth when you took that one bite of cookie that landed you right smack in the middle of a warm, gooey chocolate chip. What a bite! And the next thing you know, you're in the kitchen opening the canister and reaching in. Insert cookie in mouth, and the cycle starts all over again. Thanks to opioids, eating certain foods becomes a highly pleasurable experience, and thanks to dopamine, we're strongly motivated to eat more of those highly pleasurable foods.

It's one thing to read what happens; it's another to actually see some-one in the throes of food addiction. Watching the film *Super Size Me* brought my understanding of the matter to a whole new level. Filmmaker Morgan Spurlock ate three "super-size" meals from McDonald's every day for a month. What struck me the most while watching Spurlock's experiment was not that he gained 30 pounds or that his cholesterol skyrocketed off the charts or even that his liver became compromised. I expected those things to happen. What really stopped me in my tracks was how Spurlock began to behave. The first time he ate a super-size meal, he vomited, just like a teenager experi-menting for the first time with alcohol. But, by the end of the film, Spurlock only felt "well" when he ate the fatty, salty, starchy food from McDonald's. The rest of the time he felt depressed, washed out, irritable, and stressed; he even lost his sex drive. These are all symptoms of drug or alcohol withdrawal.

Homeostasis Gone Wrong

Now that we know about the addictive properties of foods high in refined carbs, fat, and salt, I'd like to discuss the impact of this on our country's weight and health. The bottom line is that Americans are fat because we overeat. We overeat because our diet is laden with foods containing that tantalizing combo of refined carbs, fat, and salt, which causes us to eat beyond fullness. The addictive nature of these foods is a major reason, if not *the main reason,* Americans are fat and getting fat-ter every day. In fact, some experts believe up to 70 percent of obesity in the U.S. is attributable to this issue.

We've already discussed how these foods stimulate the pleasure and reward systems in our brains. They also override the system that is sup-posed to regulate our weight. This system is called *homeostasis*—our appetites' on-off switch. When we have had enough calories for our bodies to function, the switch is supposed to turn off, leaving us feel-ing full and satiated. When our bodies require more calories, the switch flips on again, causing us to feel hungry and driven to eat. Foods with that just-right combo of refined carbs, fat, and salt—let's call them "over-stimulating foods"—actually cause the switch to malfunction. Even after we've eaten an adequate amount of calories, we continue to feel hungry.

Homeostasis has worked just fine for millions of years. So what's causing it to go haywire now? The answer is obvious: America's processed food diet. In the beginning, millions of years ago, humans hunted and foraged for food. Then we invented and streamlined agriculture, and for about 10,000 years, we humans ate a certain way. In general, our food took a pretty direct route from the farm to our mouths. But after World War II, a major shift occurred in how we ate. That's when the food distribution chain became highly industrialized. The U.S. led the charge on this initiative. One reason for the growth and expansion of the food industry in the U.S. was that factories built to crank out weaponry and war supplies were repurposed to manufacture food items once the war ended. So instead of producing tanks and bullets, factories began manufacturing frozen dinners, potato chips, and soda.

The capability to efficiently crank out a plethora of new factory food products changed not only what we ate but how we ate. Instead of eating a balanced diet of foods close to their natural state, three times a day, we began eating "fast" and "convenient" highly processed foods that bore little resemblance to the real, natural foods that humans had eaten for millennia. Today, a day in the eating life of Mr. Typical American looks something like this: Typical wakes up in the morning and for breakfast eats a couple of toaster pastries washed down with a few gulps of sugary "fruit juice." Then, at the office, he snacks on a bag of cheese puffs and a candy bar from the vending machine. For lunch, he zips through the drive-thru for a double cheeseburger, fries, and a soft drink—super-size, of course. Then it's back to the office, where he munches on whatever sweet treat his co-worker has brought in for the office—today, it's double fudge brownies. To fight the mid-afternoon doldrums, he takes a walk to the nearest coffee shop and orders his usual grande mochaccino. Then it's home to a "lean" frozen dinner of "Mediterranean chicken." Before bed, he's hit with a craving for something sweet, so he enjoys one of his favorite midnight snacks, a big bowl of Count Chocula cereal with milk. Thanks to the gobs of refined carbs, fat, and salt in Typical's diet, all day long he's been cheered on by "feel good" opioids and "eat more" dopamine.

Human beings are not biologically designed to eat this way. Is it any wonder our biological systems are going haywire?! We humans are smart, the most intelligent beings on the planet, but in so many ways we've gotten too smart for our britches. Somewhere along the way, we forgot that we don't make the rules! Mama Nature is in charge, and Mama Nature designed us to eat mostly plants, some meat when we could get it, and not all that much of either—just enough to give us the fuel we need to function. Our brains are not meant to be inundated on a daily basis with chemicals that drive us to eat more calories than we need to live.

The human body can adapt to changes in its food supply. In fact, we co-evolve with our living food supply. For instance, when cow's milk was first introduced to us about 8,000 years ago, it didn't agree with us. But in time, most of us evolved to be able to digest it. So perhaps in time, if we continue to eat great quantities of these over-stimulating foods, our brain chemistry will calm down, and not cause us to eat more calories than we need, and we won't get fat. And perhaps eating these foods will no longer give us diabetes, heart disease, and certain kinds of cancers, among countless other maladies. Who knows, maybe in time sugar will even be good for us! This, at least, is a comforting thought, right? The kicker is that this sort of adaptation doesn't happen overnight. It takes many millions of years. Since you're not going to make that train, how about continuing along with me to relearn how to eat what Mama Nature intended you to eat?

The Many Flavors of Food Addiction

Researchers have found that people react in various ways to addictive, over-stimulating foods. For some, although they will have the opioid/dopamine release when they eat over-stimulating foods, they are not prone to becoming "addicted." These are the lucky folks who can eat just one chocolate chip cookie or potato chip! These folks simply aren't programmed to overeat. For others, the cycles of opioid and dopamine release in their brains do become a problem; however, it remains purely the chemical issue that we discussed above. But for others, the problem goes a step further. It becomes emotional. You're sad, anxious, depressed. You eat a chocolate chip cookie. While you're eating the cookie, bursts of opioids are released in your brain. Opioids produced by eating over-stimulating foods can relieve pain or stress or even calm us down when we're anxious or worked up. It becomes a slippery slope, because once your emotions become part of the equation, eating takes on a new purpose: self-medication.

For still others it goes beyond the chemical reaction and the emotional self-medicating and becomes a habit. Habits develop when familiar stimuli activate pathways in your brain to produce repetitive behavior. In the case of food, over time the repetition of eating over-stimulating food creates an automatic response. For instance, at first the eating is reward driven. You know if you eat a cookie, you will feel pleasure. But if you repeat this same act often enough, it could become habit-driven behavior, less deliberate and more repetitive. When this happens, different circuitry in your brain becomes involved.

So there are various levels of food addiction:

- Chemical food addiction
- Addiction resulting from emotional self-medicating
- Habitual addiction

But also keep in mind that your reason for overeating over-stimulating foods can change depending on what's going on in your life or your environment or simply because of how your day is going. These foods are all around us, all the time. They are in our homes, at the gas station, in the vending machine or snack counter at the office, in our colleague's outstretched arms, at the street corner cart . . . you get my point. So we don't have to expend a lot of effort to acquire them and pop them into our mouths—no foraging or hunting required!

Therefore, your specific reason for eating too much of a particular over-stimulating food could change depending on where you are and what you're up to. For example, on my own personal journey, there were times when I overate because I was lonely or sad. Other times, however, I did it out of habit. For instance, once I was working on a project, and my favorite fast food at the time (frozen yogurt) was available at my favorite frozen yogurt shop on the way home from the job site. Out of habit each weekday I would go and get the extra-extra-large fat-free peanut butter yogurt with loads of sugar free hot fudge. I wasn't present for the consumption; I just wanted to get dinner (yes, at that time I considered a pound of frozen yogurt my dinner) taken care of and out of the way so I could get more work done or get some rest before I went to work the next day. In addition to this habit, I know there were times when my overeating was driven purely by an opiate/dopamine party going on in my brain. Put a dozen homemade chocolate chip cookies in front of me any hour, any day of the week, and watch the party get started! If you would like to read more about my food addition check out my previous book, *Skinny Chicks Don't Eat Salads*, which outlines my weight gain, over-exercising, emotional eating, and body image issues.

Why Do You Overeat?

In order to gain a better understanding of why you overeat over-stimulating food, and to figure out your trouble zones, I ask that you spend some time thinking and journaling about these questions. (In Chapter 11, I ask you to do journaling exercises or other "homework." Please set aside a Real-Food Notebook where you can gather information and complete exercises in one convenient place.)

- Do you believe you overeat over-stimulating food because of the chemical merry-go-round of opioid/dopamine release in your brain?

- Do your emotions ever jump in and play a role? If so, give an example of when this has happened.

- Do you ever overeat to self-medicate?

- Are there processed foods that you overeat by force of habit? If so, what are they?

- Are there any cues in your life that cause you to eat or overeat this food? If so, what are they?

Rehabbing with Real Food

So where does real food enter the equation? Well, changing to a diet of real food can actually help you lick your addiction to factory food. A diet of real food is not only healthy and a proven weight-loss strategy, it can also put you back in control of your eating. (I discuss this further in Part II: Real-Food Recovery.) In the next chapter, I show you exactly what you're up against in the factory food world we live in. The next three chapters will be a major eye-opener and will give you the complete scoop on how factory food goes from the factory farm to the assembly line to your supermarket shelf.

CHAPTER 2

Pulling the Lid Off Factory Foods

When I grow up and have kids, I want to be a mom just like Lisa Leake. Lisa's a 30-something mother of two adorable little girls. Determined to help her kids be the best people they can be, Lisa takes her job—the hardest on the planet, as all you moms can attest—very seriously. Lisa totally gets that one of her main jobs is to make sure her kids are well nourished. One afternoon a few years back, Lisa got what she describes as a loud wake-up call. It happened when she turned on *The Oprah Winfrey Show* and watched for an hour as real-food activist Michael Pollan clued her into exactly where the food she bought every week at her local supermarket came from. She was shocked and disgusted by what she learned, but most of all, she was worried for her kids and how the food they had been eating was affecting their health.

Right then and there, Lisa realized she had to make a change. Before seeing Michael Pollan on *Oprah*, Lisa and her family ate what most Americans eat. "We've always cooked a lot," says Lisa. "But our meals were often full of refined grains and sweeteners, like white flour pasta and cookies for dessert. And we ate our fair share of factory foods, like white sandwich bread, store-bought barbeque sauce, and cream of mushroom soup." Once Lisa learned how the food she and her family were eating reached the supermarket shelves, though, she stopped feeding her family a diet of factory food and began feeding them real food. (Lisa didn't make the switch overnight; that's impossible! For more about Lisa and her family's journey from a factory food diet to a real-food diet, see "Real-Foodie Lisa Leake" on page 22.)

For some, like Lisa, becoming informed about the manufacturing process is all the motivation needed to make the switch to real food. Unfortunately, this doesn't work for everyone. Just think of cigarette addiction. It's no secret that smoking causes a myriad of health problems, yet millions still smoke. Regardless of whether it will help you make the switch, it's important for you to know what goes into manufacturing the food you're taking off the supermarket shelf and putting into your body. It's an issue that has gone unexamined for far too long. Our complacency has allowed manufacturers to turn our food into perfectly engineered portions of refined carbs, fat, and salt in their effort to hijack our brains and keep us coming back for more. As a result, Americans have become overweight, unhealthy, and chemically unbalanced. It's time to pull back the lid on the food industry and get to the bottom of what you're eating.

That's the purpose of this chapter. I explain exactly what I mean by factory food and how it differs from the way we humans have "processed" our food for millennia. Then we'll take a little tour, beginning at the factory farm, proceeding to the food production plant, and ending on the supermarket shelf. After the tour, I give you a too-close-for-comfort look at the nuts and bolts of how a few of America's longtime staples are manufactured. And lastly, you'll get a little taste of the unappetizing secrets the factory food industry would rather you didn't know.

"Processed" Food: Then and Now

When I refer to factory food, I'm talking about what others call processed food. In reality, human beings have "processed" food for as long as we've been around to eat it. We've been manipulating, preserving, pickling, fermenting, and drying it for thousands of years. The difference between this kind of traditional food processing and the kind that occurs in the modern day factory food industry is that traditional food processing had two functions: *to make food easier for our guts to digest* and *to preserve it to last through tough times.* For instance, traditional bread-making neutralizes antinutrients in grains to make the minerals more available (an *antinutrient* is a substance that binds to vitamins, minerals, and enzymes to make them unavailable to the body). Fermenting cabbage to make sauerkraut increases the levels of vitamins C and B; and old-fashioned countertop yogurt preparation makes the good stuff in the milk easier to digest. Traditional food processing gave us yummy foods like sausage, cheese, pickles, and *vino!*

So how is factory food different? One of the country's foremost nutrition experts and one of my go-to real-food experts, Marion Nestle, explains it best. She says that factory foods are processed in a way that "diminishes the nutritional value of the basic ingredients; adds calories from fats and sugars; and disguises the loss of taste and texture with salt, artificial colors and flavors, and other additives."

Whereas traditional processed foods were meant to nurture our bodies and satisfy our hunger, modern factory foods end up causing us to overeat.

Not only do factory foods stimulate us to overeat, they're also full of ingredients that often turn out to be terrible for us in other ways. What's the purpose of all these additives? I mean, when you cook your own food, you add each ingredient for a specific purpose, and usually that purpose is to make the dish taste good. When it comes to factory food, are all those additives thrown into the mix for flavor? No, they're not. Just take a look at a list of reasons these additives are used, and you'll come away with a real sense of just how *unreal* these food products are. Additives are used to

- Colorize: They give your ice pop that Smurf-blue hue.
- Emulsify: Otherwise your mayo will become half water in your fridge.
- Stabilize: They make sure factory whipped cream stays foamy.
- Texturize: They give your cereal its snap, crackle, and pop.

- Bleach: They clean chicken as well as they clean your toilet bowl.

- Soften: Ever wonder why white bread has the same consistency as cotton?

- Flavor: Yum! The taste of strawberries in January!

- Preserve: You might want that candy in 20 years.

- Sweeten: A spoonful of saccharine helps the sugar free cookie go down.

In Chapter 8, I'll tell you a bit more about specific additives. For now, suffice it to say that these chemical concoctions are not what most of us think of as real food.

Not My Grandpa's Farm

I consider myself blessed to have grown up where I did. When most people think of a farm, they think of a farm like my grandparents'. It was a small operation where a host of different crops were grown and a small number of animals were raised. But the reality is that the majority of food grown in this country comes from farms vastly different from my grandparents' farm.

Most farms in the U.S. are so-called "monoculture" farms. On a monoculture farm, a single crop is grown in a large area. Monoculture farming spread in the 20th century as the mass production of food became a reality, thanks to the use of pesticides and herbicides. So what's wrong with a one-crop farm? Lots. Nature is all about diversity and balance, and no matter what we humans do, nature will always figure out how to shift things back into balance. In the case of monofarming, bugs find a way to mutate in order to become resistant to pesticides. As a result, stronger and more chemicals need to be used. Plus, the soil on a monoculture farm becomes stripped of nutrients because it's overplanted. Therefore, the food grown on a monoculture farm is not as nutritious as it should be. Lastly, the less diversity in our country's fields, the less diversity in our country's food supply. Today, according to Pollan, four crops—corn, soy, wheat, and rice—account for two-thirds of the calories we eat.

Monoculture farming extends to how animals are raised for the food industry as well. Although you might like to picture an idyllic farm complete with pigs, chickens, and cows chewing their cuds, the truth is your burger or pork chop most likely came from a *concentrated animal feeding operation,* or CAFO. A CAFO is every bit as terrible as it sounds. In a

Frankenfoods a.k.a. GMOs: Are They Harmful to Our Health?

Genetically modified organisms (GMOs) are created when a gene from one organism is extracted, modified, and inserted into the DNA of another organism. Where food is concerned, this transfer is typically made to create crops that can produce their own pesticides (kill the bugs that snack on them) or be more resistant to other pesticides (the weeds are killed but the crops are spared). Considering that it took billions of years for the current gene pool to evolve to where it is today, is it really a good idea for us to alter it? The biggest human health concern about GMOs is that the genetic alteration may cause the proteins in the food to act as toxins or allergens when consumed. Even the nutrient content of the food can be altered. Many scientists believe that research on GMOs brings up more questions than answers, and that the general public is being forced to participate in a giant experiment. The GMOs most likely to appear in either whole or derivative form in your diet are

- Soy
- Corn
- Canola oil
- Potatoes

If you want to avoid genetically modified foods altogether, buy 100 percent organic foods, as they are not permitted to contain any GM ingredients. If you can't afford to buy all organic, then limit your organic purchases to soy, corn, and potato products. As for canola oil, avoid it altogether, not only because of the GMOs involved in its production, but also because it's not a healthy fat. The same can be said for soybean and corn oils. (See Chapter 4 for more on this topic.)

CAFO, large numbers of a single kind of animal—a thousand or more in the case of cattle and tens of thousands for chickens and pigs—are kept in filthy, close, confined quarters. The animals get no sunlight or space to move around or lie down, and they're fattened up for slaughter as quickly as possible, usually with the use of hormones.

To enable them to survive in these impossible and unnatural conditions, the animals in CAFOs get a lot of help from Big Pharma. The large amounts of antibiotics they are given can lead to antibiotic-resistant bacteria, not just for the animals, but also for the people who eat them. It's simple evolution: The antibiotics kill off all but the few microbes that mutate to develop genes that allow them to survive the antibiotics. Before long, these survivors have established a drug-resistant super race, and it's possible for these harmful microbes to spread to the human population. Already, researchers have linked antibiotic-resistant strains of the pathogen MRSA to pigs raised in CAFOs.

Another concern is that the menu for animals raised in CAFOs includes food they're not designed to eat (sound familiar?). For instance, cattle are meant to graze and eat grass, but on a CAFO, they're fed soybeans and corn. And pigs, which are supposed to forage for their food, are fed just about anything, including chicken poop. (You can't make this stuff up!) The way animals are treated and what they're fed determines the nutritional value of their meat, eggs, and milk. For example, beef from pasture-raised cattle is a good source of omega-3 fatty acids. The beef of CAFO-raised cattle is not. In short, when you eat food that comes from a CAFO, you're getting fewer nutrients, and as a result of the drugs and chemicals in animal feed, you're also eating harmful toxins.

Cranking It Out

Back in the day, food was processed by artisans. Cheese and bread makers, the town butcher—these folks used traditional methods to turn raw ingredients into food that was as nutritious as it was delicious. Today, food factories crank out products that bear little resemblance to their original raw ingredients. Modern food processing techniques are designed to get us to eat faster, not better. Typically, in order to eliminate our need to chew, the food is broken down using heat and chemicals. The goop is then mixed with dyes, preservatives, synthetic vitamins, and countless other additives. Chemists and "food flavorists" in white coats work to make it as tantalizing and stimulating as possible, while tossing around lingo like "mouth feel" and "bite characteristics." To them "maximum shelf life" is factory food nirvana.

Figuring out how factory food is processed is no easy assignment. The food industry is about as forthcoming as the CIA. The reason for the secrecy is simple. If people knew exactly how the food items are made, they'd lose their appetites for them. So, more often than not, the food industry does its best to mislead consumers. After a bit of digging, though, I can share with you the nuts and bolts of how a handful of common, everyday foods are processed before landing on the supermarket shelf. I promise you'll be surprised at what's under the lids of these food items.

Cereal: Snap, Crackle . . . Extrude

Extrusion is the process used to make cereals. First, a so-called slurry of whatever grain is being used is made. (A slurry is basically a thick suspension of solids in a liquid.) The slurry is then poured into a machine called the *extruder* (is it just me, or does this sound like the name of a sci-fi villain!?). The mixture is then forced out of a tiny hole at high temperature and pressure. The shape of the hole determines the cereal's shape. A blade slices off each individual piece of cereal. The new little flake, or O, or whatever shape the cereal takes, then goes under a nozzle that sprays it with a nice shiny coating of sugar and oil. This is how cereal gets its crunch.

The major problem with the extrusion process is that it destroys most of the nutrients in the grains. It not only eliminates the fatty acids found naturally in the grains, it also obliterates the vitamins manufacturers add to fortified cereals (which is why most health claims for cereals are bogus). Plus, the amino acids naturally found in the grains are turned toxic by the process. Lysine, in particular, an essential amino acid found in grains that we need and that we must get from food because the body can't synthesize it on its own, really gets hammered by the process.

In addition to the extruding process, cereal is often loaded with added sugar as well as other additives like sodium.

Orange Juice: Freshly Squeezed Neurotoxins, Anyone?

To make factory OJ, whole oranges are put into the machine. Enzymes are added to get as much oil as possible out of the skin. Because oranges are heavily sprayed with pesticides, when the oranges are squeezed, all these pesticides end up in the juice. These pesticides, so-called cholinesterase inhibitors, are basically neurotoxins. A study carried out in Hawaii found that consumption of fruit and fruit juices was the number one dietary factor for the development of Alzheimer's disease. The researchers speculated that the real culprit was the pesticides used on fruit—and concentrated in the juices due to modern processing techniques.

One more thing about processed orange juice. Have you ever wondered why factory OJ stays cloudy, why the solids never seem to separate and settle? This is because *soy protein,* combined with soluble pectin, is added to keep the juice permanently cloudy rather than settle into layers of water, pulp, and juice, which happens naturally to orange juice when it sits. Someone who is allergic to soy might want to know this!

Bleached Flour: What Do Zits and Flour Have in Common?

Flour milled from wheat is yellow, not white. However, if it's allowed to aerate, after a month or two it will turn white. Aged flour is better for baking. That's because flour oxidizes when exposed to air over time. This strengthens the gluten bonds in the flour so you have stronger, more elastic dough. Rather than wait for nature and time to accomplish this, however, manufacturers bleach flour as a shortcut to both the white color and the better baking quality. Here in the U.S., the most common flour-bleaching agent is benzoyl peroxide. (Yes, the same benzoyl peroxide that's used to treat acne.)

Chicken Paste: Squeeze from the Bottom, Please

Giant processing plants go through a lot of chicken in a day. After removing the parts that we buy in the supermarket—breasts, thighs, wings, and drumsticks—they're left with a heap of scraps that aren't salable. But nowadays, thanks to new industrial techniques, edible connective tissue can be separated from this scrap heap, mashed into a mound of pink chicken paste, and used to make a myriad of chicken-like products such as chicken nuggets and hot dogs. Processors are allowed to use ammonia to kill bacteria and, because it tastes horrible, it's artificially flavored to . . . well, to taste like chicken! Then, the off-putting pink color is dyed away. Foods made from chicken paste must be labeled "mechanically separated chicken" (the same process is used with turkey, too). It just goes to show that one man's heap of chicken scraps is another man's frozen chicken patty.

I hope that after reading this chapter you have a better understanding of where the food you buy in the supermarket comes from. My intention is not to gross you out or make you afraid to eat cereal or drink OJ but to get you thinking about how the food items you throw into your cart are manufactured. If, after reading the chapter, you're ready to swear off factory foods and fully embrace real food, great! But the most important takeaway is that now you can't plead ignorance. The food choices you make will be better informed ones—always the best kind!

Real-Foodie Lisa Leake: 100 Days of Real Food and Beyond!

Lisa Leake is one of my favorite real-foodies. Lisa is a pretty, 30-something mother of two adorable girls. She's brilliant, warm, funny, and, when it comes to taking care of her family, completely fearless. What's so fantastic about Lisa is that once

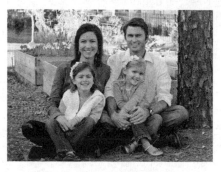

she made up her mind to make the switch from factory food to real food, she got to work to make it happen. But that's just the half of it. As she did the research, played label detective, and experimented with new foods and recipes, she realized that the process she went through to make the switch for her family might help others do the same. For that reason she launched a blog to share her experiences with others.

After a few months of blogging about making the switch to real food, she decided to do something big, something bold, something to encourage as many other people as possible to commit to making this important change. The result was a pledge that she and her family took to eat only real food for 100 days. To share her family's journey, she launched her fabulous blog, www.100daysofrealfood.com. One of her first posts was the "Real Food Charter" that her family would adopt. Her family's real-food rules were set down after much research and thought. For example, they vowed to eat only locally raised meat, and in moderation. Another role was that her family would eat only 100 percent whole wheat, whole grain bread. A third rule was that her family would eat lots of fruits and vegetables, which they would buy at their local farmers' market as often as possible. After accomplishing their goal and eating real food for a total of 100 days, the family decided to take on another challenge: 100 days of real food on a budget. Again, Lisa shared her family's experiences on her blog, helping others in the process. In addition, Lisa now writes a column about making the switch from factory food. It appears in about two dozen major national newspapers, including the *Miami Herald*, the *Sacramento Bee*, the *Kansas City Star*, and the *Los Angeles Times*. Here's Lisa's story in her own words.

At the beginning of 2010 our eating habits were probably just like those of any other family. We felt like we were making fairly healthy food choices, although we certainly weren't following any special rules. For instance, we didn't think twice about eating bottled salad dressings or many overly processed foods, or where the meat sold in our grocery store meat department came from, or how our milk was processed. Then came the *Oprah* show "Food 101 with Michael Pollan." After the show, [my husband] Jason and I both decided to read Pollan's book *In Defense of Food*, which ended up being life changing for us. As it turned out, a lot of what we thought were "healthy" food choices were actually just what the food industry was labeling as "healthy" and not good choices at all.

Jason's background is fairly different from mine. As a young child he lived with his parents and aunts and uncles on a hippie commune in Oregon. They grew and raised all of their own food. Jason and his parents have since become more industrialized when it comes to eating, but that doesn't change their basic understanding of where our food comes from. On the other hand, as a child I had both Doritos and Kraft Macaroni & Cheese as staples in my diet, and I barely stepped foot on a farm. This shaped my views as an adult. As most other wives and moms can relate, the woman of the house often does the meal planning and food shopping, therefore I was (and still am) the biggest influence on our family's food choices. And after reading *In Defense of Food*, I decided it was time for some big changes to those food choices. It wasn't easy at first, but we slowly revamped everything from what we bought, to where we shopped, to how we cooked. For instance, we stopped eating white bread, and began eating only 100 percent whole wheat bread; we began shopping at our local farmers' market and eating loads of fresh fruits and veggies; and we cut out all soft drinks, and began drinking only water, natural fruit juices, coffee and tea (and for the adults, vino and beer!). (To see the family's other "Real Food Rules," see www.100daysofrealfood.com/real-food-defined-a-k-a-the-rules/.)

It has been such an eye-opening experience for us, one that's been full of surprises. By far the biggest of which were the changes that we experienced to our health. We changed our diets because we thought it was the right thing to do. The fact that my daughter's constipation and asthma cleared up, my husband and I lost a few pounds, and that I had much more energy were all bonuses for us.

CHAPTER 3

Sugar's Bitter Side

Ah, the 90s. What a decade. All us kids were listening to grunge bands, wearing flannel, and watching *Friends*, *Seinfeld*, and *The X-Files*. Everything was neon, colorful, and "totally radical!" Everyone, including *moi*, was rocking the Jennifer Aniston haircut, boasting about going to music festivals like Lollapalooza, and secretly doing the "Macarena" in our living rooms. Good times. But when I think back on the 90s, what I mostly recall is that it was my Decade of Sugar.

I was a hardcore sugar addict. My sugar binges were epic. I remember one Sunday afternoon at my grandparents' house when I wolfed down an entire pecan pie and chased it with a family-size bag of Doritos. It was back then that I concocted what I still to this day consider the sugar fix to end all sugar fixes. Here's how it went down: My absolute favorite cereal growing up was Golden Grahams. Inspired by the Rice Krispies Treat (of which I was also a big fan), I whipped up a batch of Golden Graham Treats! Same marshmallowy gooeyness of a Rice Krispies Treat, but Golden Grahams instead of Rice Krispies. Genius, right? And I wasn't afraid to mix it up. My lowest points were when I'd mix frozen Cool Whip with peanut butter; after topping the result with about a dozen packets of Equal, I'd dive in with a spoon. (In gourmand-speak, this creation was my Sweet-Dusted Cool Peanut Mousse.) I'd often joke that I was "addicted to sugar." Today, I know it was no joke!

Even though I was raised on a farm, surrounded by amazing real food, when I was responsible for feeding myself, I went for processed food. I didn't even give it a second thought. There wasn't a distinction between "real" and "factory" food back then. Back then, food was whatever you bought at the supermarket, and that happened to be fake food. When I look back on the girl I was then, I see someone who was unhealthy, overweight, and downright out of control. And, quite frankly, ignorant. Sure, I knew I wasn't exactly eating "healthy," but at the same time, I honestly didn't realize the hold that sugar had on me, or understand the health risks and consequences of my terrible eating habits.

In this chapter, I share the information about sugar that I wish I had then. First I'm going to tell you, point blank, what's wrong with sugar, and then we'll take a look at how our country's diet became so full of it. After a frank discussion about how sugar compromises our health, we'll figure out how it fits into a real-food diet.

What's Really Wrong with Sugar?

I'm sure this isn't the first time you're hearing about the harmful effects of sugar; it's a warning you've likely heard hundreds of times from dozens of sources. Maybe you're even become inured to the fact that sugar is a major culprit behind a long list of health issues. That's why I want to take it a step further, and talk about what's *really* wrong with sugar.

First, let's go over why we're even talking about sugar. It's delicious, it makes anything taste good, and it gives us a terrific burst of energy when we eat it. How can something so good be so wrong? The answer to that question has two parts. First and foremost, what's wrong with sugar is how much of it we eat. Today, Americans eat an average of 170 pounds of sugar per person every year—including high fructose corn syrup. That's a lot of freakin' sugar! The second part of the answer is that, biologically, human beings are not designed to eat that much sugar.

While much has changed since humans lived in caves, one thing that hasn't changed is the system we have in place to provide our cells with the fuel they need to function. This system is set up to process the same kinds of foods that our cavemen ancestors ate: fresh fish, a great source of proteins and essential fatty acids; the meat of animals that grazed on a variety of plants; and foraged nuts, berries, and edible shrubs that grew in mineral-rich soil. These cave folk did eat sugar-containing fruit, but that sugar came in a neat package with vital nutrients and fiber that

Digesting Sugar: The Slower, the Better

To understand why it's important for sugar to be digested slowly, you have to understand what happens when sugar is introduced into your body too fast. Here's the rundown: When you eat a glazed donut, for instance, a tidal wave of glucose (sugar) crashes into your bloodstream, causing your blood sugar levels to immediately skyrocket. As a result, insulin gets to work clearing your bloodstream of the glucose and distributing it to the cells in your body. If those cells don't need it, the glucose gets stored as fat.

The problem is insulin does its job too well; it's so quick to clear the glucose from your bloodstream that your blood sugar levels fall too low too fast, and your brain panics and screams for more glucose. That's why about an hour after eating that donut you find yourself obsessed with finding another sweet treat. So you grab a bag of Oreos or a Twinkie and the cycle starts all over again. Because your cells have all the glucose they need, the glucose gets stored as fat. And despite the calories you're taking in, you never seem to achieve a feeling of fullness or satisfaction, and you're constantly craving more sweets.

Note that this vicious cycle is triggered only when we eat large quantities of sugar and other refined carbohydrates. If you eat smarter, say an egg-white omelet and a slice of whole-wheat toast, the glucose your body craves will be slowly released into your bloodstream, kind of like a time-release capsule. Your brain would then be content with the slow, steady stream of glucose coursing through your bloodstream and it won't feel the need to switch into panic mode and convince you to seek out more sweets.

slowed the absorption of the sugar into the blood (the slower the break-down, the better). And occasionally, cave grandma or grandpa stumbled upon honey and, after going head to head with a few angry bees, they enjoyed a really fantastic treat. But those instances were few and far between.

All in all, sugar made up a very small percentage of our ancestors' caloric intake. The point I really want to drive home is that our bodies simply aren't genetically programmed, nor do they have the adaptive ability, to healthily handle 35 times more than the amount of sugar our ancestors ate. Not to mention the fact that the sugar we are eating today is a far cry from the sugar they ate. We're certainly not eating 170 pounds of natural honey and fruit sugars that come with gobs of vitamins and minerals.

America's Sugar High

Christopher Columbus first brought sugar to America, igniting what was to become a national sweet tooth. For centuries throughout America's history, sugar and other sweeteners like honey and molasses were used to make delicious desserts like Martha Washington's Currant Cake, Boston Cream Pie, and the Depression Era "Mystery Cake," popular because it required very few ingredients during a time when everything was scarce. By the mid-20th century, the typical household dessert consisted of pie, ice cream, or some kind of pastry. We would have been fine had it all stopped there, with sugar a once-in-a-while treat or as a dessert after a healthy meal, but in the 1970s, food preparation reached an all-new sugar high. That's when the factory food industry learned to create and mass-produce high-fructose corn syrup.

High-fructose corn syrup is a super-cheap sweetener that has become the predominant sweetener in soft drinks and in many processed foods. However, the proliferation of sugary factory foods can't be entirely blamed on the invention of HFCS. The truth is, the food industry most likely would have increased the production and marketing of sugary foods with or without it. After all, whether a candy bar is sweetened with HFCS or with refined sugar from sugarcane, it causes the same cycle of addictive eating with the same result for the food industry—increased sales.

"Sugar" comes in several different forms. Typically, when folks are discussing refined sugar, they're talking about

- **Sucrose**: common table sugar. During digestion it breaks down into glucose and fructose. Sucrose is found in many plants, but is extracted for table sugar primarily from beets and sugarcane.

- **Glucose**: the primary sugar in the blood. The fuel the brain runs on.

- **Fructose**: the primary sugar in fruit. Today, most sugary factory food products are made with either sucrose or fructose, often in the form of high-fructose corn syrup.

I know the whole sucrose/fructose thing can be really confusing, so let me break it down for you: Sucrose is made up of 50 percent fructose and 50 percent glucose. HFCS is made up of fructose and glucose in a ratio of either 55/45 or 42/58. (High-fructose corn syrup isn't particularly high in fructose, but was so named to distinguish it from ordinary glucose-containing corn syrup. As you can see, one commonly used version of the ingredient, HFCS-42, actually contains less fructose than table sugar.)

Some researchers contend that fructose—and therefore HFCS—is the cause of increasing rates of obesity; however, there's no hard and fast scientific proof of this. Chemically, however, as you can see, table sugar and HFCS are very similar. They're both fructose and glucose. So I consider all the hype about one being better or worse for you than the other to be misguided.

At the end of the day, both sucrose and HFCS end up as glucose and fructose in the body, both are rapidly absorbed carbs, both are common ingredients in factory food, and both contain calories devoid of nutritional value. If HFCS is the culprit behind the obesity epidemic, it's most likely just because we're eating too much of it. Whereas we once ate sugar only as part of our dessert, now you can find sugar—in a multitude of forms—in breakfast foods, snacks, frozen meals, condiments, soft drinks, boxed rice or pasta dinners, canned goods, and many more items.

So if Americans are so hopped up on sugar, why isn't everyone walking around in a jolly good mood? This is an important question, and the answer further highlights the drawbacks of a sugar-filled diet. At first blush, it may seem that, since eating sugar causes a sharp increase in the pleasure chemicals in your brain, you'd walk around feeling fabulous as long as you kept eating it. Well, most of us know from firsthand experience that this isn't how it works.

Brain neurotransmitters are finite, meaning that once you run out, you have to manufacture more. If you don't eat the foods necessary to make more, you will feel terrible sooner or later no matter how much sugar you eat. The nutrients that allow you to replenish neurotransmitters are found in real foods, not in nutrient-deficient sugar. So why doesn't your brain crave those foods? It's only focused on its immediate needs, which is always going to be glucose, because that's the primary fuel for our brains. So the brain fixates on sugar, often to the exclusion of real foods.

Sugar and Health

Sugar—whether it's table sugar or HFCS or organic, unbleached cane sugar—is basically calories with zero nutritional value. Sugar is what's considered a *simple carbohydrate*. A simple carb is made up of one or two sugars. (Remember that HFCS is made up of fructose and glucose.) Besides sugar, other simple carbs are polished white rice and refined white flour. These simple carbs have been stripped of vitamins and fiber. The manner in which they're refined extends their shelf life mainly because it renders them less nutritious to pests.

After the food industry removes the best parts, only the carb or starch is left. Basically, our bodies treat all of these simple carbs the same, so the same problems that arise with sugar also occur with white rice, white flour, and other simple carbs. That's because a simple carb is devoid of the vitamins and minerals necessary to digest and metabolize itself, so our bodies end up depleting vitamins and minerals from our diet or from internal stores in order to digest it. For instance, if you eat a lot of simple carbs and don't eat a lot of foods that contain B vitamins, you'll become depleted of B vitamins. If this happens, you might begin to suffer from a burning sensation on your tongue, wrinkles surrounding your lips, exhaustion, gastrointestinal problems, thinning and graying hair, and the blues.

Sugar also depletes antibodies, which fight viruses, bacteria, and yeasts. We've already discussed how simple carbs make us overeat, contributing to weight gain and obesity. They also cause bone loss and tooth decay. Simple sugars aggravate asthma, cause mood swings, provoke personality changes, contribute to mental illness, worsen nervous disorders, promote the growth of gallstones, hasten hypertension, and cause arthritis.

But the most serious health problem by far occurs because simple carbs raise the body's insulin levels. As described earlier, excess insulin promotes the storage of fat and contributes to high blood sugar, triglycerides, and cholesterol, leading to obesity, diabetes, and heart disease. High insulin levels also inhibit the release of growth hormones, which in turn depresses the immune system.

Sugar in a Real-Food Diet

The good news is consumers are becoming aware of the health and weight issues surrounding sugar. The bad news is the food industry views this as an opportunity.

First, let's talk about sweeteners. One of my clients came to me very excited one day after discovering a wall of "natural" sweeteners in a health food store. She had gotten it into her head that instead of buying sugary fake foods to satisfy her sweet cravings, she could now simply learn to bake her own sweat treats using any one of the number of "natural," "organic" sweeteners for sale at the health food store. Surely, "unrefined dehydrated cane juice" was a healthy alternative to white table sugar, she thought. As you may have already guessed, she was wrong. The food industry is stamping labels like "natural sweetener" and "organic" on refined sugar in the hopes that consumers will fall for the ploy.

But the fact is, it's like putting lipstick on a pig. No matter what wholesome-sounding verbiage is stamped on the package, your body is still going to recognize it for what it is: sugar. So products like "organic cane sugar," "raw sugar," and even molasses, brown sugar, and maple sugar are all going to have the same negative health effects as table sugar or HFCS. That's because they're all simple sugars. And you might be surprised to learn that honey also falls into the simple sugar category because 96 percent of the dry matter in honey is simple sugars: fructose, glucose, and sucrose. No wonder the honey bear is the only animal found in nature with tooth decay (honey decays teeth faster than table sugar). In fact, honey has the highest calorie content of all sugars, with 65 calories per tablespoon compared to the 48 calories per tablespoon found in table sugar.

Now let's talk about another food industry ruse. Many products that are appearing in health food stores are full of sugar but disguised as healthy, such as gummy bears with added vitamins and herbs. I also came across a box of fruit snacks made with "real fruit juice from concentrate." Also on the ingredient list was "evaporated cane juice." Both ingredients are, yep, you guessed it, simple sugar. So be aware and be smart. Candy is candy. Sweets and desserts are sweets and desserts, not nutritious food. A good rule of thumb is that if an ingredient ends with "syrup" or "-ose," it's a sugar; if it's honey or fruit concentrate, it's still sugar.

So where does sugar fit into a real-food diet? Eating a real-food diet doesn't mean you have to forever forgo the pleasures of sugar. Life is about living, and you should enjoy the many pleasures of life—one of them being a right-out-of-the-oven chocolate chip cookie. But you don't want to enjoy yourself right past a state of good health. Sugar is not poison, but it is best eaten in small doses. My rule of thumb is to limit processed sugars to the occasional dessert or celebration. This might sound right to you, or it might sound as though I've lost my mind. If you're in the latter camp, don't panic; once we begin exploring the possibilities of a real-food diet, you'll come to learn that this rule is really a piece of cake—uh, carrot.

Real-Foodie Vin Miller:
A Better Way

The best word I can think of to describe real-foodie Vin Miller is "brilliant." No one is more knowledgeable about real food and living a healthy lifestyle than Vin. Vin initially decided to make the switch from a factory food diet to a real-food diet for health reasons. But real food soon became his passion and his life's work. An avid real-food blogger at www.naturalbias.com, Vin is currently working toward a master's degree in nutrition. Vin's going to tell you a bit about himself in his own words:

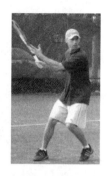

"As a child, I was often sick and frequently suffered from stomach pain and headaches. It certainly didn't help that I ate a lot of processed foods and was frequently exposed to second hand cigarette smoke. As a result, I began adulthood with a predisposition for poor health. College life certainly didn't help matters. My diet continued to be just as poor as it had always been, my sleep schedule became much more irregular, and like most college students, I was having more than just a few drinks on weekends. As I became more and more fatigued, I began to question if something was wrong, but having never experienced vibrant health, I didn't know what I was missing and accepted the fatigue as normal. Despite living a healthier and more regimented lifestyle after college, I was still pushing through life more so than enjoying it. Getting out of bed was a major ordeal nearly every morning, and after a typical workday, it seemed like a tremendous effort just to drive myself home.

On one such drive home, I vividly remember being so fed up with my exhaustion that I was on the verge of deep depression. After questioning why the basic activities of life seemed to be so difficult, I berated myself for being weak and concluded that if everyone else can deal with it, I can too. Despite my frequent exhaustion, I still forced myself to exercise and play sports as often as I could manage. Although these were some of my favorite activities, which helped to keep me sane, forcing myself to be physically active when I didn't have the energy undoubtedly made things worse. I frequently experienced what is commonly referred to as an exercise hangover, which intensified many of my symptoms and left me even more tired than normal for a number of days, sometimes longer.

Ultimately, I sought medical help. After a lot of back and forth between different practitioners, tests, time and money, and frustration, test results indicated a number of hormone imbalances including adrenal fatigue, nutrient deficiencies, and viral infections. I was diagnosed with chronic fatigue syndrome. And because I had been bitten by a tick in a highly endemic area, the specialists suspected Lyme disease as the primary problem.

I followed the treatment prescribed by my medical team for nearly a year, and during that time, I continued to educate myself on how to support my recovery through healthier lifestyle habits. I was impressed by the center's thorough testing and advanced knowledge of chronic illness, but was beginning to question their treatment approach. Although they described their approach as natural and holistic with minimal use of drugs, they were neglecting a number of important lifestyle factors and I was also displeased with the large number of supplements and prescription medications I was taking. Throughout most of the treatment, I was taking more than 60 pills every day, and each time I discussed one of my symptoms with the doctor hoping to shed some light on the cause of my problems, I would be given a new prescription.

By the time a full year had passed, I had made some notable improvements, mostly as a result of my lifestyle changes, but overall, wasn't feeling much better than when I had started. I was frustrated by my lack of progress and had a strong suspicion that I was heading down the wrong path. Inspired by the knowledge and confidence I gained through my own research, and more notably, my frustration with the medical community, I decided to discontinue the treatment and rebuild my health on my own. That's when I decided to change my eating habits and fully embrace a real food diet. For me, eating a real food diet meant that I would give up refined carbs and factory food and eat a diet of mostly vegetables and fruit, and as much as possible, free range chicken and eggs, grass fed meat and dairy from grass fed cows. In addition, I would eat food that was locally farmed and raised, and organic when I believed it was appropriate. Deciding to discontinue the intensive treatment for chronic fatigue syndrome and Lyme disease and take my health into my own hands was one of the best decisions I've ever made. As a result of my hard work and dedication, I now feel better than ever, have eliminated the majority of my symptoms, and have more energy, physical capacity, and resistance to illness than a large majority of the population. Even though I still have room for improvement, I feel like a new person with a new life and none of this would have been possible without the ambition and determination to find a better way."

CHAPTER 4

The Skinny on Fat

When I work with clients who are making the switch from a factory food diet to a real-food diet, time and again the biggest hurdle for them is to get over their fear of real fat. Folks are terrified of butter, lard, coconut oil, the skin of a chicken, whole milk, and the list goes on. I harbored the exact same fears until I made the switch myself. Like many Americans, I was afraid that eating this food all but guaranteed I would get fat and sick.

As I mentioned earlier, when I enrolled in culinary school to pursue my lifelong passion for cooking, I was terrified. I knew full well when I signed up to learn to cook traditional French cuisine that copious amounts of butter and other fat were going to be part of the deal. However, that reintroduction to real fats, along with other real foods, turned out to be the beginning of my real-food epiphany. As I did my research into real food, I was shocked at just how wrong I had been about fat. Everything I had always believed to be gospel about fat was not only wrong, but completely backward.

The reality is that the fats we've been warned to steer clear of are actually vital for our health. On top of that, the fats the food industry has promoted as lifesaving alternatives to unhealthy, artery clogging fats are actually the ones that are detrimental to our health. My hope in this chapter is to once and for all set you straight on fats. I know how confusing it all seems when you first delve into it, so I'm going to take you down the same trajectory I took to get my essential fat facts. First, we'll take a look at how things got so mixed up in the first place. Then I'll lay everything out straight for you—what kind of fat is good for you and what kind of fat is detrimental to your health. Lastly, we'll take a peek inside the fat factory.

How Fat Became the Villain

Fat gets a bad rap. Unfortunately, people associate the fat we eat with the fat on their guts, while completely dismissing the reality that fat is an important macronutrient that our bodies need to function. Before we go another step further, let's first take a look at the role fat plays in how our bodies function.

- In the human diet, fats from animal and vegetable sources provide us with a concentrated source of energy; the building blocks for cell membranes; and the building blocks for a variety of hormones and hormone-like substances such as prostaglandins that regulate many of the body's functions.

- Fats slow down nutrient absorption so that we can go longer without feeling hungry.

- In addition, they act as carriers for important fat-soluble vitamins A, D, E, and K.

- Fats in the omega family are called "essential" because our bodies can't produce them; we must get them from foods. And we need them! Our brains rely on omega-3 fats; a deficiency causes depression, among other maladies.

- Dietary fats are needed for the conversion of carotene to vitamin A, for mineral absorption, and for a host of other processes.

So fat isn't a tantalizing guilty pleasure; it's actually an important nutrient that we need to function. However, despite its importance in our diet, fat has been cast as the villain, accused of clogging our arteries and expanding our waistlines. The reason for fat's bad rap is that for years government recommendations, medical doctrine, the food industry, and health experts have encouraged us to eat low-fat and fat-free foods, cautioning people to avoid fats in general and saturated animal fats in particular. In place of saturated fats, the "experts" have recommended partially hydrogenated oils, claiming that they reduce the risk of heart disease. These folks held up margarine, for example, as a healthier alternative for the heart than butter. So saturated fats, like butter, were the villains, while factory fats, like margarine, were the lifesavers.

Where exactly did this notion come from? The issue can be traced back to the 1950s to a researcher named Ancel Keys, whose Seven Countries Study became the basis for his claim that cardiovascular disease was primarily the result of high serum cholesterol levels brought on by a diet high in saturated fat. Keys's claim was called the "lipid hypothesis." The lipid hypothesis is an unfortunate example of strong researcher bias affecting research results. For his part, Keys was bound and determined to prove his lipid hypothesis. He basically cherry-picked the data he used to support it. Subsequent independent analysis of the data Keys used shows that he picked only those countries with numbers that supported his hypothesis and omitted a significant amount of data that showed there was actually no correlation among saturated fat, cholesterol, and arteriosclerosis. But this information has been largely ignored. Part of this can be explained by powerful industry groups with a vested interest in having his theory accepted as fact. Part of it can also be attributed to Keys' strong and persuasive personality.

Whatever the reason, the result is that today, some 50 years later, a lipid hypothesis based on faulty data is accepted as true by governments, health organizations, the media, and the food industry, and we, the general population, are left eating a recommended diet that is causing more harm than good. While this thinking is now beginning to change as new research comes to light, change comes slowly to the establishment. After all, if low-fat and fat-free is a healthier way of eating, why are we, as a society, getting fatter and sicker? Since the early 1980s, the consumption of red meat, butter, and other sources of the evil villain, saturated fats, are down, while consumption of carbohydrates and poly-unsaturated fats has skyrocketed. Simultaneously, the incidence of obesity has risen to epidemic proportions, and rates of diabetes have increased dramatically.

Real Fats

Once I let my fat fear go and began to do my research, I uncovered some pretty surprising facts about the stuff. Check this out:

- Lard and bone marrow are rich in monounsaturated fat, the kind that lowers LDL and leaves HDL alone. (HDL is considered "good cholesterol" and LDL is considered "bad cholesterol.")

- Stearic and palmitic acid, both saturated fats, have either a neutral or beneficial effect on cholesterol.

- Coconut oil, a saturated fat, fights viruses and raises HDL.

- Butter is an important source of vitamins A and D and contains saturated butyric acid, which fights cancer.

- Researchers have uncovered that a substantially greater absorption of carotenoids occurs when salads are consumed with full-fat than with reduced-fat salad dressings.

- Putting butter on a rapidly absorbed food like bread, which is made of white flour, a simple carb, will cause it to be absorbed more slowly into the bloodstream rather than in one quick burst.

So what kinds of fats are "real," and fit in with a real-food diet?

The answer is that all the traditional fats—that is, fats that have been used for generations by home cooks and haven't been harmfully altered in a factory—are healthy and fit into a real-food diet. This includes butter, lard, coconut oil, sesame oil, and olive oil. (In Part III, we'll go into way more detail about the individual cooking oils, so stay tuned!)

These fats are primarily saturated or monounsaturated. It's no accident that, like with most animals, the fat that exists in your body is mostly either saturated or monounsaturated. In fact, only 4 percent of your fat composition is polyunsaturated. So when you're giving your

Fat Chemistry

Three kinds of fats exist in nature, each with a unique chemical makeup.

Saturated Fats

Found predominantly in animal fats and tropical oils like coconut oil and in lesser amounts in all vegetable oils, saturated fats are structured so that all available carbon bonds are occupied by a hydrogen atom, which makes them highly stable and also straight in shape, so that they are solid or semi-solid at room temperature. Saturated fats are less likely to go rancid than other kinds of fats. In addition, when heated for cooking, they DO NOT form dangerous free radicals as other types of fats do.

Monounsaturated Fats

The monounsaturated fats most commonly found in our food is oleic acid, the main component of olive oil and sesame oil as well as the oil in almonds, pecans, cashews, peanuts, and avocados. Chemically, monounsaturated fats are structured with one double bond, composed of two carbon atoms double-bonded to each other. Because this bond causes the molecule to bend slightly, these fats do not pack together as easily as saturated fats, so they tend to be liquid at room temperature but become solid when refrigerated. Like saturated fats, however, monounsaturated oils are relatively stable. They do not go rancid easily and can also be used in cooking.

Polyunsaturated Fats

Polyunsaturated fats have two or more double bonds. The two polyunsaturated fatty acids found most frequently in our foods are linoleic acid, with two double bonds (omega-6), and linolenic acid, with three double bonds (omega-3). (The omega number indicates the position of the first double bond.) Because your body cannot make these fatty acids, they are called "essential" and must be obtained from foods. Polyunsaturated fatty acids have bends or turns at the position of the double bonds and hence do not pack together easily. They remain liquid even when refrigerated. Unpaired electrons located at the double bonds make these oils highly reactive. When they are subjected to heat or oxygen, as in extraction, processing, or cooking, free radicals are formed. It is these free radicals, not saturated fats, that can contribute to the causes of cancer and heart disease. For that reason, factory-processed polyunsaturated oils, such as corn, safflower, soy, and sunflower oils, should be strictly avoided.

body traditional fats, you're giving it what it needs to be healthy. However, because of the unnaturalness of CAFO farming, the saturated fat found in these animals is no longer the healthiest choice. When it comes to animal fat, fats from grass fed, pastured, and wild animals—butter, lard, beef tallow—are as real and healthy as it gets. When it comes to oil from plants, the oil must be cold pressed and unrefined;

Real-Food Diet Fat Do's and Don'ts

Traditional, Healthy Fats: Do!

ANIMAL FATS

Fats from grass fed cattle, sheep, bison, and other livestock

Butter and cream from grass fed cows

Lard from pastured pigs fed a natural diet

Egg yolks from pastured chickens

Fish oils, especially cod liver oil

VEGGIE OILS

Cold-pressed extra-virgin olive oil

Cold-pressed unrefined flaxseed oil

Wet-milled unrefined coconut oil

Cold-pressed unrefined macadamia nut oil

Cold-pressed unrefined walnut oil

Cold-pressed unrefined sesame oil

MODERN INDUSTRIAL FATS: DON'T!

All hydrogenated and partially hydrogenated oils, including lard from CAFO-raised animals

All veggie oils when refined or heated such as corn, safflower sunflower, and soybean oils otherwise, it's not a healthy choice. See the list below of what I consider to be healthy, REAL fats. You will notice that the majority of vegetable oils sold in supermarkets today are absent from the list. Most vegetable oils are what I consider "factory fats," primarily (but not always) polyunsaturated fats. These unstable oils are highly sensitive to oxidation and rancidity. In fact, the oils often actually go rancid during the process of making them! Food manufacturers then have to deodorize and bleach the oils to make them edible.

I don't count fat grams or the percentage of calories from fat. However, like most things, it's best to eat real fats in moderation. So while I don't want you to obsess over the number of fat grams you're eating, I'm not giving you license to gorge on foods that contain delicious real fats. And the reality is that for weight loss and weight maintenance, it's important to be mindful that of the three macronutrients (proteins, carbs, and fats), fats contain the most calories per gram. Proteins and carbs have 4 calories per gram, while fat has 9 calories per gram. And when we eat too much fat, our bodies convert it to fat storage. But the good news is that the body burns traditional, real fats much faster than it does factory-produced trans fat or partially hydrogenated fat, which our bodies tend to store for a rainy day.

So how much fat do I recommend? Although this is not a book about calorie counting, I think it's important for you to have general guidelines. When your goal is to lose weight, your fat intake should be around 30 percent of your total diet. That works out to no more than 40 grams of "real-food" fats per day (10 grams per meal). As for the times when you're simply aiming to maintain your weight, I recommend that you eat no more than 50 grams of healthy, traditional fats per day. And I suggest that you eat a variety of traditional fats and oils. Remember that each has its own specific and fabulous health profile, so variety is the key.

The Essentials

Essential fatty acids are fats that our bodies cannot make, so we have to get them from the food we eat. There are two essential fatty acids humans need: omega-3 and omega-6, both polyunsaturated fats. Most likely you've heard all about omega-3. And you probably know that you can get it in fish (such as salmon), fish oil, cod liver oil, and red meat (especially from grass fed animals).

What exactly do you gain from consuming omega-3 fatty acids?

- Lower blood pressure

- Improved insulin sensitivity (and therefore lower blood sugar)

- Increased total HDL

- Decreased overall possibility of heart disease

- Decreased cardiovascular inflammation

- Improved mood

- Improved fertility, and the development of a fetus to a healthy size

- Improved neurological function in general, including memory and ability to learn

Sounds good, right? But here's the glitch: Omega-6 fatty acids are the counterparts to omega-3. We're designed to eat a specific balance of omega-3 (found in fish and animals) and omega-6 (vegetable fats). The problem is that we're not anywhere close to even. We're getting way too much omega-6 (from the copious amounts of partially hydrogenated vegetable oils in the processed foods we eat), and too few omega-3. Some experts consider the imbalance to be as great as 20 to 1. Ideally, the ratio should be at 2 to 1 (omega-6 to omega-3). And it would be best if we got our omega-6 fatty acids from unprocessed seeds and nuts rather than from processed vegetable oils.

It's not that omega-3 fatty acids are inherently good and omega-6 fatty acids are inherently bad; it's simply that we've created a problem through a lack of balanced eating. It's important that we get our omegas back in balance! Eating too much omega-6 and too little omega-3 causes clots and constricts arteries, which increases the risk of heart attacks, increases swelling that worsens arthritis, and aggravates a skin disease called psoriasis. It may block a person's ability to respond to insulin, causing high insulin and blood sugar levels and obesity. It increases hormone levels of insulin-like growth factor 1, which causes certain cancers.

Here's the solution: Eat more meat (grass fed when possible), fish, eggs, coconut oil, and butter (especially from grass fed cows). Avoid foods that contain margarine, vegetable shortening, and vegetable, corn, safflower, soybean, sunflower, and canola oils.

The Bad Fats: Factory Fats

You've had the good news; now the bad. As we've already discussed, for years, medical experts, government agencies, and medical organizations urged Americans to stop eating traditional saturated fats, and to opt instead for partially hydrogenated oils in order to reduce the risk of heart disease. For example, they held margarine up as healthier for the heart than butter. Now, a large body of scientific research shows that these altered fats actually increase cholesterol and the risk for heart disease.

Why Vegetable Oil Is Bad for You

Because of the lipid hypothesis, the "experts" have told us to replace saturated fats with so-called "polyunsaturated vegetable oils" (sometimes referred to as "polyunsaturated oils" or POs)—vegetable oils manufactured by the food industry, such as corn, soybean, sunflower, and canola oils. In addition, a huge percentage of processed foods contain vegetable oils. There are two reasons to avoid these oils. One, as I've already mentioned, is that POs are high in omega-6 fatty acids, so eating too much of them causes an imbalance of omega-6 and omega-3. While both omega-6 and omega-3 are essential, it's just as important to get these nutrients in the right ratio. Otherwise, you can be setting yourself up for major health problems, as I mentioned before.

The other reason has to do with how the factory vegetable oil is processed. Here's the lowdown: Grains, beans, and seeds are crushed under high heat and extracted with chemical solvents like hexane, which is then boiled off. The oils may then be bleached, refined, and deodorized. All of these processes damage the polyunsaturated fats within the grains, beans, and seeds, destroy vitamin E, and create free radicals. Many experts believe this processing is what causes the oil to be associated with heart disease and cancer.

Just a word here to avoid confusion between "polyunsaturated fats" in general and "polyunsaturated oils" specifically: The polyunsaturated fats in grains, beans, and seeds are perfectly okay. The fat is tucked within the grain, seed, or bean in its real, natural form as polyunsaturated fatty acids (either omega-3s or omega-6s). It's when this fat is pulled out and manufactured into polyunsaturated oil that it's turned into a substance that is detrimental to our bodies.

Cooking with Real Fats

An important quality of every fat is its ability to withstand heat in the kitchen. Some fats are appropriate for heating, others are less than ideal, and some are downright unacceptable. Heavily saturated fats, which tend to be solid at room temperature, are best for heating; monounsaturated fats are second best; and polyunsaturated fats, which are liquid at room temperature, are ideally used cold.

Below are some great tips to help you match the best real fat with your cooking needs:

Roasting and sautéing

Use butter, coconut oil, or lard (from grass fed and pasture raised animals), which are mostly saturated or monounsaturated. Chiefly monounsaturated oils, like olive and macadamia nut, are the next best choice for cooking. However, you need to avoid heating these oils to the point that they smoke. Olive oil, good for sautéing, is actually not suitable for high heat cooking. A good blend for sautéing is half butter, half olive oil. Sesame oil, which contains more polyunsaturated fat, is less suitable for cooking but still acceptable.

Vinaigrettes and other cold dressings

Use flaxseed, olive, or walnut oil.

Trans Fats

As if that weren't bad enough, factory vegetable oils are also "hydrogenated" to make more solid, longer lasting products like vegetable shortening and margarine. To make margarine or shortening, high temperature and pressure are used to extract the oil. After this process, any oil still remaining in the seed or grain is removed with hexane solvents. Then the oil is steam cleaned, a process that removes all the vitamins and antioxidants but, of course, leaves behind the solvents and pesticides. Next, the oil is mixed with a nickel catalyst and put into a huge high-pressure, high-temperature reactor. Hydrogen gas is forced into the oil at high pressure in a process known as hydrogenation. What goes into the reactor is a liquid, but what comes out is a semi-solid that looks like gray cottage cheese and smells terrible. Emulsifiers are mixed in to smooth out the lumps. The product is steam cleaned a second time to get rid of the horrible smell. Then it is bleached to get rid of the gray color. And finally, you have vegetable shortening.

To make margarine, processors add artificial flavors and synthetic vitamins to vegetable shortening. Because manufacturers aren't allowed to add a synthetic color to margarine, they add a natural coloring called "annatto." The not-butter-but-made-to-look-like-butter is then packaged in blocks and tubs. For years, this stuff has been promoted as a healthier alternative to the saturated fats humans have thrived on for millennia. And because it is longer lasting than butter, it's a primary ingredient in processed baked and fried foods like chips, crackers, cookies, and cakes. In the process of hydrogenation, the fatty acids in the oil become transformed by hanging on to some of the hydrogen. This in turn makes the oil much denser. If you fully hydrogenate, you create a solid out of the oil. But if you stop partway, you end up with a semi-solid or "partially hydrogenated oil" that has a consistency like butter. Because it's cheap, this partially hydrogenated oil is a big favorite as a butter substitute among food manufacturers.

However, unlike butter, hydrogenated oils contain high levels of trans fats. Trans fats are fatty acids that have been "transmogrified" by high-heat processing and are found inside partially hydrogenated oils, so if

Weston Price: Granddaddy of the Real-Food Movement

In 1932, Dr. Weston Price, a Cleveland dentist, launched an investigation after becoming increasingly concerned about the declining health of his patients. Observing rampant tooth decay and crowded and crooked teeth, he noted that people with these dental problems always suffered from other health problems as well. Dr. Price believed these problems were not hereditary but nutritional. He was beginning to doubt that the diets his patients were consuming, which were based on sugar, white flour, and vegetable oils, were resulting in good health.

Having heard that isolated societies that ate only local foods had pristine dental health, Dr. Price spent more than 10 years traveling to remote parts of the world studying the health of populations untouched by Western civilization. His goal was to discover whether nonindustrialized societies were healthy and, if so, what they were eating. He visited secluded villages in Switzerland, Gaelic communities in the Outer Hebrides, indigenous peoples of North and South America, Melanesian and Polynesian South Sea Islanders, African tribes, Australian Aborigines, and New Zealand Maori. In all, Price found 14 different societies that enjoyed beautiful, straight teeth with no decay, as well as fine physiques and resistance to disease, just as long as they followed their traditional diets. Dr. Price also discovered that whenever these traditional societies began to eat Western foods, physical degeneration followed. Health problems showed up immediately, and structural defects (namely, narrow jaws and crooked teeth) appeared in the next generation. Plus, widespread obesity often accompanied the transition to modern factory foods.

Although Dr. Price is no longer with us, his work lives on with the Weston A. Price Foundation, a nonprofit founded in 1999 to disseminate the his research. The foundation is dedicated to restoring nutrient-dense foods to the human diet through education, research, and activism. For anyone interested in making the switch from factory food to real food, the foundation's Web site has an amazing amount of fantastic information: www .westonaprice.org.

you read a label that says "partially hydrogenated oil," you know the product contains trans fats. So what's the problem with trans fats? While the fatty acid itself becomes transformed chemically, it retains its ability to pass into the body and take up the job of an untransformed fatty acid. So it's like a fatty acid body snatcher! For instance, fatty acids anchor to our cell walls and act as gatekeepers for stuff going in and out of our cells. Trans fatty acids can get away with impersonating these gatekeepers. But once they're at their post, they completely screw up their job by allowing foreign invaders to pass into cells or not letting necessary supplies in.

At the end of the day, trans fats are terrible for you. Studies show that, for one thing, they work to increase LDL, the "bad" cholesterol, and they also decrease HDL cholesterol, the "good" cholesterol. There is also evidence to suggest that trans fatty acids may accumulate in the body, because the digestive system has difficulty figuring out what to do with them.

I hope this chapter has succeeded in clearing up any confusion or misconceptions you might have had about fat. Factory fat—including refined vegetable oils like corn, safflower, sunflower, soybean, and canola as well as trans fats like margarine and shortening—is a major contributor to the health and weight crisis in this country. The real tragedy is that for so many years, consumers honestly believed they were making healthier choices when choosing these fake fats over traditional real fats. The lesson is that the responsibility for how you nourish your body is truly in your hands. The buck really does stop with you, and the stakes are super-high.

PART II

Real-
Food
Recovery

CHAPTER 5

What Is "Real Food"?

So what is real food?! That's the trillion dollar question. The very fact that we have to ponder such a question goes to show how far removed we have become from our food sources. Here's the thing: If you're looking for a checklist, you've come to the wrong place. The fact is, it's up to each of us individually to make choices about what we consider "real" food. If I were to present a long, detailed list here of can-eats and can't-eats, quite frankly, some of you in certain parts of the country would not have access to all of the foods on the list.

I divide my time between Los Angeles and New York City, and even in these major cities there are many items designated as "real foods" by real-food advocates that are difficult to find. So if you can't get ahold of a grass fed ribeye or a free range pork chop, does that mean you can't eat meat? Or if you can't afford to shop at a grocery store that sells expensive organically grown peaches, does it mean no peaches for you? No way! That's not what a real-food diet is about. The fact is, we have to work within the reality we live in. We can't all pick up and move to a farm and grow and raise our own food. But we *can* get informed and make thoughtful decisions based on that information.

Don't worry; I'm certainly not going to leave you on your own in the ridiculously complicated realm of today's food distribution system. I'll give you some general suggestions that I hope will help you to devise your own personal Real-Food Charter. (An exercise in Chapter 11 will also help you do this.)

My Real-Food Guidelines

Here is my personal definition. Real food

- Is as close to its natural state as possible.
- Is not overly processed and does not contain more than five ingredients (This is Michael Pollan's general rule, and I think it's a winner.)
- Has no harmful artificial additives or preservatives.
- Contains no added sugar.
- Contains no refined carbs, such as white flour or high-fructose corn syrup.
- Contains no factory processed polyunsaturated oils.
- Contains no hydrogenated vegetable oils.
- Contains zero trans fats.
- Is 100 percent whole wheat and whole grain.

Below is a list of what I call "if possibles." If it's possible for me to buy my real food in this state, I do. If I can't, I buy the next best thing. (Look for much more on this topic in Part III.)

If possible, buy:

- Produce and animal products that are locally grown and raised
- Beef that is grass fed, antibiotic-free, and hormone-free
- Pork that is antibiotic-free, hormone-free, and free range
- Chicken that is antibiotic-free and free range
- Eggs from chickens that are antibiotic-free and free range

Real-Foodie Mark Bittman: Rock Star

I was a fan of real-foodie Mark Bittman well before I began my real-food journey. Mark is a long-time contributor to the *New York Times* and the author of several outstanding cookbooks. Since the late 1990s, Mark wrote *The Minimalist* column for the *Times*, which regularly inspired all of us to cook, eat, and love food. From the beginning of his career as a food writer, Mark strove to battle the ascendance of factory food and a general decline in food quality. He has been on the front lines of the food movement. In January 2011, he published his last column in order to take on a new challenge. Now, in addition to his continued writing for the *New York Times Magazine* and a column in the paper's Opinion section, Mark is also blogging for the *Times*. Mark's new platform gives him the opportunity to cover the exciting food revolution that's under way in the U.S., a revolution that he himself helped bring about.

Like Vin Miller, Mark made a big change in his eating habits after dealing with health issues, including high cholesterol and sleep apnea. As chronicled in his most recent book, *Food Matters: A Guide to Conscious Eating*, Mark improved his health and lost weight by shifting his diet to emphasize vegetables, legumes, and beans over meats and processed food, which helped him reach his weight and health goals without resorting to rigid dieting or calorie counting. Mark allows himself a little meat at dinner.

I asked Mark his opinion on the question "What is real food?" He replied, "I think that people should be moving more in the direction where they rely more on plants and less on everything else in their diet. [M]ovement in that direction is what's going to make people eat better and I hope cause some changes in the way our food system works."

- Dairy from antibiotic-free, grass fed cows
- Produce and animal products that are organically grown, *if appropriate* ("Certified organic" often isn't what you think it is. See Chapter 9 for more about what "organic" means in today's food marketplace.)

These are the guidelines I have developed on my own journey from a factory diet to a real-food diet, and my hope is that they will help you wherever you are on your journey. If you're just getting started, you'll figure out that the more you learn and immerse yourself in the real-food community where you live, the more your own, very personal guidelines will take shape. For many of you, weight loss is your number one priority in switching to a real-food diet, and it is the reason you picked up my book. In the next chapter, I serve up a real-food diet for weight loss. Follow this eating strategy and you will lose weight. For real!

CHAPTER 6

Real Food Equals
Real Weight Loss

Tiffany, a fellow culinary student and a client of mine, is what I refer to as a "repeat offender." A real stunner, Tiffany is tall with dark hair and lovely blue eyes. When she began her dieting roller coaster, she had just become engaged. With only 10 months until her wedding and 20 pounds to shed, Tiffany embraced a popular weight loss program. With her type A, goal-oriented personality, she succeeded in losing 25 pounds in 8 months. So Tiffany's problem wasn't losing weight; it was *keeping the weight off* once she switched from diet mode to real-life mode.

Once she was back in real-life mode after her wedding, Tiffany gained back those 25 pounds in just a matter of weeks. So back into diet mode she went, eating frozen diet meals and drinking diet soda. As before, Tiffany dropped the pounds, and again, just like before, as soon as she switched back to her real-life eating habits, she gained them all back and then some. Over the next few years, Tiffany found herself losing and gaining weight over and over and over again. During that time, she cycled through Weight Watchers, the Atkins Diet, and the South Beach Diet, and even resorted to sheer starvation while taking the popular diet pill Xenadrine. After losing 20 pounds through starvation, she quickly gained them back.

I met Tiffany between her diets, when she was one of my classmates at Westlake Culinary Institute. After learning that I was a nutritionist, she approached me about nutrition and weight loss. She confided in me about her past as a serial dieter. When I asked her what her diet was like these days, she replied that she was pretty much eating on the go. Because of her busy schedule with work and school, she just had no time to cook, except when she was at culinary school (how ironic). On a typical day, she'd have a large Starbucks cinnamon dolce latte, with extra sugar-free syrup, and an oversize blueberry muffin for breakfast; lunch was usually a frozen meal of some kind (Lean Cuisine or Weight Watchers) or a meal deal from the nearest fast-food joint. And dinner was a takeout affair: pizza or chicken parmigiana from the Italian place, sweet and sour chicken from the Chinese place, or enchiladas, rice, and beans from the Mexican place. Every once in a while her husband would cook (and let's just say he wasn't famous for his prowess in the kitchen). Just last night, she told me, he had made Hamburger Helper—the macaroni and cheese kind—and a salad topped with his favorite Wishbone Fat-Free Thousand Island dressing. She also confessed that between meals she had been visiting the vending machine at her office. But she did try to go with a "healthy" option, like a chewy cinnamon and raisin granola bar. And she sipped on Mountain Dew pretty much all day long. So, despite her passion for food and cooking, in her everyday life she was essentially eating processed food wherever and whenever she could get it.

In the past, I would have sat down with Tiffany and personalized a diet plan for her. I would have worked around her lifestyle, choosing healthier alternatives to what she was eating. For instance, instead of a giant Starbucks muffin for breakfast, I would have recommended a cup of low-fat yogurt and an egg white omelet. For lunch and dinner, I might have set her up with a meal service I used for my busier clients. And to keep her blood sugar stable, I would have recommended that she eat two snacks a day, such as a snack bar with a good ratio of protein to carbs or a small handful of chocolate covered pretzels. To replace her Mountain Dew, I would have suggested a diet soft drink.

But that day I took a different track. I looked at Tiffany and I knew it was time to do something different—for her as a client and for me as a nutritionist.

"Okay, Tiff," I said. "Are you tired of yo-yoing with your weight?"

"So tired!" she replied.

"Are you tired of eating packaged 'diet' food?"

"Beyond tired! I'm such a foodie, and it haunts me constantly."

"What if I showed you a way to eat that would not only get the weight off, but allow you to eat *real food*, no more fat-free, sugar free, fake factory food. Real food that will help you lose weight, keep it off, *and* get you to a place where you're super-healthy?" I said.

"Count me in," she said.

"But what if I told you that it would require a bit of effort on your part, would you be willing to commit? And Tiff, you're going to have to tie on an apron and get into your home kitchen—no more excuses that you don't have time to cook at home. I know you love to cook, you are in culinary school, for cryin' out loud! No more grab-and-go eating!" I said.

"Okay, I'm in," she said, a bit more reluctantly than before.

And that's when I began to share with Tiffany what I had recently learned about real food and its fat-melting powers. I loaded her up with reading materials, including all of Michael Pollan's books, Nina Planck's *Real Food: What to Eat and Why,* and Sally Fallon's *Nourishing Traditions.* Then, over the next month, I met with her regularly in my office and talked with her in class about her diet whenever possible. Together we went to the farmers' market, Whole Foods, Trader Joe's, and the regular supermarket. We even ferreted out real-food choices at Walmart and Costco. In addition, we visited health food stores and the local co-op. We even took a road trip to an organic farm. Tiff's journey turned out to be as much a learning experience for me as it was for her.

Within about 3 weeks, Tiffany was completely off fake food and was eating only real food. Three months after Tiffany first visited my office, she had shed 20 pounds. All while attending culinary school! Even more importantly, she reported feeling better than ever. I myself noticed that she had a new vitality about her that she hadn't had before. Perhaps best of all, she had developed a much healthier relationship with food—real food. Previously, she had relegated food only to the culinary school part of her life. Part of her feared food much the same way I had when I first started culinary school (remember my butter terror). Now she began to see real food as what she needed in her real, day-to-day life to nourish her body, mind, and spirit. And whereas previously she had convinced herself that she had "no time" to cook, now she embraced cooking, and even started a real-food dinner club with her friends. At the same time, I made sure she had a repertoire of no-cook strategies for eating real food as well. As for me, I decided then and there that it was time to upgrade my practice and began giving my clients the option of adopting what I had begun to refer to as my real-food weight loss diet.

How a Diet of Real Food Leads to Weight Loss

In the first part of this book, you learned the difference between a diet of overly processed food and a diet of real food. Plus, you've been shown the health dangers of eating a factory food diet. Now, it's time to focus on the weight loss possibilities of eating a real-food diet. I believe that the modern factory food diet is to blame for the majority of our country's weight problem. Before 1900, obesity was an extremely rare condition, as were diabetes and heart disease. For most of human history, obesity was all but unheard of.

If you switch from a processed food diet to a real-food diet, you *will* lose weight. Period. Even if your primary goal in eating real food isn't weight loss but general health (as it was for our real-foodie Vin Miller) or family concerns (as for Lisa Leake), once you rid your diet of addictive fake foods, you will lose weight without even trying. However, if weight loss is your primary goal (as it is for most of my clients), my surefire strategy of eating real food is specifically designed to help you to shed pounds. This chapter takes you step-by-step through my real-food weight loss plan.

So how exactly can eating a real-food diet lead to weight loss? First, you'll be achieving balance in your diet, eating the optimal mix of foods on a regular schedule. Second, when you stop eating processed foods, you remove from your diet added sugar, refined carbs, refined salt, and harmful additives and preservatives that contribute to weight gain and stand in the way of weight loss. Finally, when you start eating real food, you add two key nutrients—fiber and omega-3 fats—that help you shed pounds more quickly. To sum it all up in three Real-Food Diet Rules:

1. Eat a protein-carb or fat-carb combo every 4 hours.

2. Avoid added sugars, refined carbohydrates, refined salts, and harmful additives and preservatives.

3. Consume fiber and omega-3 fats every day.

Rule #1: Eat a Protein-Carb or Fat-Carb Combo Every 4 Hours

One major reason you lose weight on the real-food diet is that you will strike the right balance when you dish up a plate of real food. There are two main components to that balance: (1) making sure you're eating the right combinations and proportions of carbs, proteins, and fats; and (2) munching on real food every 4 hours.

PROTEINS, FATS, AND CARBS . . . OH MY!

You now have a good sense of what constitutes real food. Now it's time to put it all together on your plate and chow down.

There are three macronutrients: protein, fat, and carbs. Fat and protein are essential to the structure and functioning of our bodies. As for carbs, our bodies use them for energy. If we don't need the energy immediately, insulin ensures that surplus carbs are stored as body fat, a little security against starvation during lean times. Because they don't cause insulin to rise as quickly, dietary fat and protein are less likely to be stored.

This doesn't mean that carbs are bad for you per se. In fact, they're necessary to feel happy and to not feel hysterically hungry. However, as I described in Chapter 3, simple carbs like refined sugar, white flour, and white rice enter the bloodstream rapidly, leading to blood sugar spikes and other unhealthy consequences. Complex carbs, on the other hand, must first be broken down into simple carbs, so blood sugar rises slowly. The fiber in complex carbs further delays the spike in blood sugar. Examples of healthy complex carbs are

- Fruit
- Grains
- Kefir
- Legumes
- Milk

- Nuts
- Seeds
- Starchy veggies*
- Yogurt

To ensure that you have balanced blood sugar levels throughout the day, it's important that your meals have a balance of the three macronutrients. As a general rule, you should obtain about 20 percent of your calories from protein, 50 percent from complex carbs, and the remaining 30 percent from real, healthy fats.

But don't worry. You don't need to do a lot of calculating and figuring to reach those proportions. An easier rule to remember: Make sure that each of your meals includes a complex carb and a protein or fat. Proteins and fats naturally lower the rate of the release of sugar from carbs into the bloodstream. So eating these foods in combination helps stabilize blood sugar, prolong satiety, and make weight loss much easier. A typical protein-complex carb combo (or PC combo) meal is grilled wild salmon with brown rice. A fat-complex carb combo (FC combo) meal might be a simple snack such as chilled organic dates with a small handful of raw almonds or green olive tapenade spread onto 100 percent whole wheat crusty bread. You can also eat a combination of all three, such as scrambled eggs with whole wheat toast or lean grass fed steak with a side of steamed broccoli and a sweet potato with a small pat of butter.

*Examples of starchy vegetables are acorn squash, beets, butternut squash, corn, green peas, leeks, lima beans, okra, parsnips, potatoes, rutabaga, sweet potatoes or yams, and turnips.

MUNCH REAL FOOD EVERY 4 HOURS

In addition to eating the right combination of real food, eating every 4 hours is the best way to keep blood sugar levels balanced and avoid food cravings. If you're eating to lose weight, *when* you eat is just as important as *what* you eat. When it comes to losing weight, people are confused; they think they should eat less food, less often. Many people who have tried to lose weight have adopted the unwise strategy of skipping a meal or two and dramatically slashing calories, thinking food deprivation is the ticket to weight loss. They couldn't be more wrong!

Having a bite to eat every 4 hours, whether it's a full-on meal or a snack, will keep your blood sugar at a consistent level. If you eat only when you are ravenously hungry, that means you've waited until your body is out of stored glucose. When that happens, your blood sugar level is at an all-time low and you'll feel it. You'll lose your ability to concentrate, you'll feel light-headed and you'll likely experience physical hunger pangs. Ouch! When this happens, you won't instinctively grab for a plate of real food. Your brain will work hard to convince you to pig out on easily digested carbs. It'll want fuel, and fast! You'll have set yourself up to crave all the foods you shouldn't eat. It will be difficult to resist the urge to visit the office vending machine. To avoid this, simply have a bite every 4 hours; your blood sugar will love you for it and you'll set yourself up to choose the right foods.

Portion Control

Although you may be eating more often than you're used to, that doesn't mean you should be eating more overall! I'll talk more about portion control in the real world in Chapter 11. Until then, I want to make it clear that when I use the term "portion control," it does not mean that you will be eating tiny portions or going hungry! Not at all! You'll just be making better choices and setting yourself up for success rather than failure.

Rule #2: Avoid Added Sugar, Refined Carbs, Refined Salt, and Harmful Additives and Preservatives

When you make the switch to a real-food diet, you avoid the pitfalls that make fake factory foods addictive, fattening, and unhealthy. And for an added bonus, removing the above ingredients from your diet will result in better overall health.

LOSE THE REFINED SUGAR AND CARBS AND LOSE THE WEIGHT

Losing weight on a real-food diet is also aided by what you're *not* getting on your plate: refined carbs. As we've already discussed, refined sugar and all other refined carbs are major ingredients in nearly all factory foods, and today they're being consumed in record proportions. In the early 1800s, the average American consumed about 12 pounds of sugar per year. According to USDA statistics, by the year 2000 the average consumption of sugar, including corn sweeteners such as high-fructose corn syrup, increased to more than 170 pounds per person! Now, remembering that refined carbs act the same as sugar in our bodies, add in the large amount of other refined carbs we eat, such as white bread, white rice, and white flour, and the prevalence of obesity and poor health isn't all that surprising. In Chapter 3, you learned about the prevalence of both sugar and refined carbs in factory food, but now it's time to gain an understanding of how they affect weight gain.

Consider this: In laboratory studies, squirrels, when given the choice between acorns and chocolate cookies, take the cookies every time. Why is this? The exact same reason that we humans are so hooked on refined sugar and carbs. During the course of evolution, squirrels and humans rarely encountered large quantities of concentrated, high-energy foods like refined sugar and refined carbs. Our food preferences evolved and enabled us to survive in forests and African savannas, where animals were lean and fibrous. Food shortages were a fact of life, and sugar came only in the form of ripe fruits and honey, which were available only on an intermittent, seasonal basis. As a result, our food selection mechanisms don't include protections against overeating sugars. So today, both animals and humans lack brakes for runaway junk food cravings.

As I've already discussed, addiction to refined carbs and refined sugar has made Americans overweight. It's also the reason so many of us can't seem to lose weight or keep it off once we've lost it. Refined carbs like white rice and those used to make white bread, pasta, and refined sugar have had most of their fiber and nutrients stripped away. They turn into blood sugar (glucose) so fast that they cause a spike in our insulin levels as soon as we eat them. The insulin spike is followed by a drop in blood sugar levels, which leaves us feeling tired and hungry and wanting to eat more. The unfortunate result of this scenario is that

A Word about Pasta

As you may have noticed, I'm Italian. And as you can probably guess, I was raised eating and loving pasta. So you're likely wondering where I stand on pasta. Here's the deal: Remember in Chapter 2 when we spoke about the difference between "traditional" versus "factory" food processing? How the two are different in that factory food processing diminishes flavor and nutrition, while traditional food processing enhances both? Well, Asians and Italians have been processing wheat flour, eggs, salt, and water into pasta for thousands of years. The result has been a fiber-rich, vitamin B-rich food that's healthful and, I must add, delicious! But just as with cheese, yogurt, and other traditional foods, the factory food industry has hijacked pasta. Today, not only are many brands of pastas on the supermarket shelves not made the traditional way, they are also void of nutrients and full of pesticides from over-sprayed wheat fields.

The good news is there are several delicious organic brands of pasta on the market that are made in a more traditional manner. I recommend eating 100 percent whole wheat pasta until you've met your weight loss goals. It has fewer calories, and the whole wheat slows down the digestion of the pasta. One of my favorite brands is Bionaturae whole wheat pasta, sold at Whole Foods and other health food stores. I find it to be succulent and delicious, never grainy or dry. Other great brands include Barilla, Barilla Plus, and Whole Foods' 365 Everyday Value Organic Whole Wheat Spaghetti. Grandma and Grandpa Avanti would approve!

it makes us want to eat more refined carbs. When we do, we start the cycle all over again.

THE PROBLEM WITH SALT

Salt is not evil. In fact, salt is essential to life. Human blood plasma and lymphatic fluids have a composition similar to that of ocean water. Salt and water comprise the inorganic or mineral elements of your body and play a specific role in the functioning of cells. Salt helps carry nutrients into cells and pump waste materials out. It helps regulate blood pressure and fluid volume, keeps the pressure balance normal in the lining of the blood vessels, and is necessary for the absorption and digestion of food. Three million years ago, Stone Age humans got the salt they needed from eating bloody meat, fish, and sea vegetables.

The problem with salt is that Americans eat too much of it. Research connects too much salt with high blood pressure. Nearly 80 percent of the salt in American diets is hidden in the processed food we buy in stores or in restaurant food. Next to refined sugar and refined carbs, refined salt is the most seductive ingredient in factory food. As with refined sugar and refined carbs, the food industry deploys salt as an ingredient to hook you with and keep you coming back for more.

A diet of real food is the best way to take back control of your salt intake. According to both the American Heart Association and the Department of Nutrition at the Harvard School of Public Health, healthy adults should consume less than 1,500 milligrams of sodium per day. Unfortunately, most individuals consume more than 3,000 milligrams per day, according to the Harvard School of Public Health. By the USDA's reckoning, a food is low in sodium if it contains no more than 140 milligrams per serving. (FYI: Although many people use the terms "sodium" and "salt" interchangeably, sodium is actually the ingredient in salt that can lead to health problems. Forty percent of salt is sodium; the rest is chloride and other elements.)

On the real-food diet, you'll find you don't need much salt because real food is already bursting with flavor. When you do use salt in your real-food kitchen, however, I recommend that it be sea salt. Typical commercial table salt is an industrial leftover. First, the chemical industry removes the valuable trace elements of salt, then heats it to 1200°F. We get what's left, which is sodium chloride plus industrial additives including aluminum, anticaking agents to keep the salt pouring smoothly, and dextrose. The dextrose stains the salt purple, so it is then bleached. Unrefined sea salt is 82 percent to 84 percent sodium chloride; the rest is other good stuff, like calcium magnesium and more than 80 trace elements including iodine potassium and selenium, all nutrients that have vital functions, among them maintaining a healthy fluid balance and replenishing electrolytes lost in sweat.

HOW ADDITIVES AND PRESERVATIVES
CAN SABOTAGE YOUR WEIGHT LOSS

There's a great deal of research that connects certain additives and preservatives to potential health issues, as we've already discussed. But what about the link between additives and preservatives and weight management? Although the research continues to be debated, there have been studies that link HFCS and trans fat to weight gain. For instance, in 2010, a Princeton University research team demonstrated that all sweeteners are not equal when it comes to weight gain: Rats with access to high-fructose corn syrup gained significantly more weight than those with access to table sugar, even when their overall caloric intake was the same.

Similar conclusions have been reached regarding trans fat—that foods containing trans fat make you gain more weight than eating foods containing other fats with the same number of calories. In addition, researchers at Wake Forest University have found that diets high in trans fat lead to a higher distribution of weight around the abdomen, a situation that leaves folks more vulnerable to a variety of health risks.

Add monosodium glutamate, or MSG, to the list of additives that might be playing a role in making Americans fat. Researchers found that people who eat more MSG are more likely to be overweight or obese. And the increased risk wasn't because folks were overeating, according to the research conducted at the Gillings School of Global Public Health, University of North Carolina at Chapel Hill. The link between high MSG intake and overweight held even after accounting for the total number of calories people ate. MSG is one of the world's most widely used food additives. It's found in processed foods from chips to canned soups. In the latest research, published in the *American Journal of Clinical Nutrition*, scientists followed more than 10,000 adults in China for about 5.5 years on average. Men and women who ate the most MSG (a median of 5 grams a day) were about 30 percent more likely to become overweight by the end of the study than those who ate the least amount of the flavoring (less than half a gram a day), the researchers found. After people who were overweight at the start of the study were excluded, the risk rose to 33 percent.

So, three harmful additives have already been connected to weight gain. What about the slew of harmful additives and preservatives that haven't been researched in this context? My gut tells me if three of the most commonly used additives might be helping to make us fat, then most likely there are others out there doing the same. Another important reason to avoid additives and preservatives that are already suspected of harming our health is that when you feel good and are healthy you have an easier time losing weight, and eating fewer additives can make you feel and be healthier, setting you up for successful weight loss.

Rule #3: Consume Fiber and Omega-3 Fats Every Day

The real-food diet features these two key nutrients that have been shown to help you shed the pounds. Make sure you eat them every day!

FIBER AND WEIGHT LOSS

When you eat a diet of real food, you can stop worrying about whether you're getting enough fiber in your diet. That's because real food is loaded with fiber. Dietary fiber is the part of whole grains, vegetables, fruits, and nuts that resists digestion in the stomach and intestines. This indigestible fiber was the main component of the hunter-gatherer diet. Nuts, seeds, roots, and other plant materials that are hard to chew or digest kept primitive humans' digestive systems working overtime.

A daily intake of 20 to 35 grams of fiber is a great ballpark to shoot for, not only for weight loss, but for all of the other health benefits fiber has to offer. Most Americans who eat a factory food diet get only 10 to 15 grams of fiber per day, but if you eat a real-food diet, you should have no trouble reaching your goal. Examples of fiber-rich foods include

- Brown rice
- Fruits (especially high in fiber are fruits with skin, such as apples and pears)
- Legumes (lentils, dry beans, and peas)
- Veggies
- Whole grains

Today, studies show that a fiber-rich diet is a crucial factor in weight management. Fiber by itself contains no calories, but it provides the bulk in your diet that gives you the satisfaction of chewing and the feeling of being full. Fiber has several other perks that help you control your weight. For example, foods containing fiber take longer to eat, which means your stomach feels full sooner and you eat less. Due to its greater fiber content, a single serving of whole grain bread can be more filling than two servings of white bread. Fiber also moves fat through our digestive system faster so that less of it is absorbed.

There are two types of fiber: water-insoluble and water-soluble. Water-insoluble fiber, found in vegetables and whole grain breads and cereals, adds bulk to the diet. These fibers do not dissolve in water, so they pass through the gastrointestinal tract relatively intact, and speed up the passage of food and waste through your gut. In addition, water-insoluble fiber adds bulk to our stool so that we actually feel the urge to go to the bathroom. Like every other muscle in our bodies, our bowels need exercise, and going to the bathroom regularly is the best way to get a bowel workout. Without water-insoluble fiber, the bowels do not get enough exercise, leading to fewer bowel movements and constipation. Hemorrhoids can also result from a deficiency of water-insoluble fiber due to the strain bowels need to exert when they don't get enough exercise. Water-insoluble fiber also aids the growth of gut bacteria, organisms that eat sugars and fiber and prevent the proliferation of bad bacteria that can make us sick.

Below is a list of foods high in water-insoluble fiber.

- Avocados
- Beans
- Broccoli
- Brussels sprouts
- Cabbage
- Carrots
- Chickpeas (garbanzo beans)
- Eggplant
- Greens (such as collards, kale, and turnip greens)
- Mushrooms
- Peas (such as black-eyed peas and green peas)
- Peppers
- Potatoes with skin
- Pumpkins
- Rhubarb
- Spinach
- Sweet potatoes (with skin)

On the other hand, water-*soluble* fiber, found in fruits, seeds, and oat products, exits the stomach more slowly, causing you to feel fuller longer. Water-soluble fiber absorbs fluids as it moves through your digestive track. During the process, the fiber dissolves, thickens, and forms a gel. This gel binds with cholesterol from the liver and carries it out of your body through your waste. Your body has to pull cholesterol from your bloodstream to restock, reducing your blood cholesterol (a good thing!). The gel moves slowly through the digestive system, delaying the release and absorption of sugar, thereby moderating blood sugar levels.

Below is a list of foods high in water-soluble fiber.

- Apples
- Avocados
- Bananas
- Berries (such as blueberries, blackberries, and raspberries)
- Dried fruits*
- Guava
- Kiwi
- Oranges
- Pears

*Examples of dried fruits are plums, figs, raisins, apricots, and dates. They are best eaten in small quantities; however, dried fruits are high in sugar and often contain chemicals added to keep them looking attractive.

To review, shoot for a daily intake of 20 to 35 grams of fiber, containing both (1) water-insoluble fiber, which adds bulk to your diet that makes you feel fuller longer, and (2) water-soluble fiber, which helps balance your blood sugar and keeps you from feeling hungry.

Vegetables and fruits with skins are what I consider the A-Team of high-fiber foods. That's because they're so high in nutrients and don't come with the baggage of other fiber sources like whole grains. Meat and dairy products contain no fiber, and refined grains have had most of their fiber removed. While whole (unrefined) grains are a good source of fiber, many people have allergies to grains because the gluten in them is one of the hardest proteins for humans to digest. Even folks who aren't gluten-intolerant are at risk of having health issues with whole grains. Phosphorus in the bran of whole grains is stored in the grain within a substance called phytic acid. Phytic acid combines with iron, calcium, magnesium, copper, and zinc in the intestinal tract and blocks the absorption of these vital nutrients. Whole grains also contain enzyme inhibitors that can interfere with digestion.

But there is a super-easy remedy that will enable you to eat whole grains without worrying about getting a bellyache (this does not apply to people who are gluten intolerant or who have any kind of allergy to whole grains!). Traditionally, people usually soaked or fermented their grains before eating them. Doing so neutralizes troublesome phytic acid and enzyme inhibitors, and in effect predigests grains so that all their nutrients are more available to you. Even many people who are allergic to grains can tolerate them well when they are prepared this way. To enjoy whole grains as part of your real-food diet, simply soak them for at least 7 hours and up to 24 hours before cooking or baking with them. Here are a few easy predigestion tips.

- Soak whole grains such as oats, barley, millet, and quinoa in warm water (2 cups of water per 1 cup of grain) with a couple of tablespoons of lemon juice in a warm, dry place.

- Soak ground corn in water with a pinch of baking soda when making polenta, grits, or corn bread.

- Soak rice for an hour and dried beans overnight with a pinch of baking soda.

Adding fiber to your diet will help you lose weight and improve your health, but do it gradually. A rapid increase in consumption of fiber may result in gas or diarrhea. And be sure to drink plenty of fluids when adding fiber to your diet. Eight glasses of liquid a day are recommended because fibrous foods draw water from the intestines. While fiber is normally helpful to your digestive system, without adequate fluids it can cause constipation. A floating stool and easy passage indicates that your diet has enough fiber.

OMEGA-3 FATS AND WEIGHT LOSS

The other ingredient you'll get in your real-food diet that will inevitably lead to weight loss is omega-3 fats. As I noted in Chapter 4, most folks who consume a processed food diet do not get adequate amounts of this vital nutrient. Omega-3 fats, such as those found in fresh fish, can help prevent obesity, diabetes, and heart disease.

Here's how: Omega-3 fats regulate blood sugar levels and burn fat. In particular, DHA and EPA (two of the most common omega-3 fats) are directly involved in activating the genes that control fat metabolism. For instance, mice fed fish oil are leaner than those fed the same number of calories from corn oil. Another reason omega-3 fats are so helpful when it comes to weight loss is that they help stabilize insulin levels and suppress the appetite. So, unlike sugar and refined carbs, which make you want to keep eating, omega-3 fats make you put on the brakes! They stabilize blood sugar levels, helping you resist the food cravings and hunger pangs that low blood sugar causes. As you learned in Chapter 3, a diet too high in refined carbs frequently causes low blood sugar.

Other benefits of omega-3s are improved kidney function and the alleviation of depression. Omega-3s improve your kidneys' processing of fluid waste, which cuts down on bloating and water weight. And if you've ever suffered from depression, you know it can stand in the way of weight loss. When you're depressed, or even just feeling down, you may be tempted to self-medicate with foods that stimulate your pleasure center—in other words, sugary and fattening factory foods. Omega 3s help increase the levels of serotonin (the happy chemical) in the brain. This not only helps you feel better (without the unhealthy addiction to sugary foods!) but also increases your energy. We all know how important energy is to our motivation to exercise, not to mention to shop for and prepare real foods.

So by eating more omega-3s, you mitigate depression, increase energy, improve kidney function, stabilize blood sugar levels, and suppress appetite—all vital to any weight loss program. At this point, you're probably thinking, "Okay, I'm in; so where and how do I get these fabulous fatty acids?!"

The best way to get omega-3 fatty acids is to eat fatty fish two or three times a week. In fact, almost all seafood, including shrimp, crabs, and oysters, contains omega-3s. Why are fish and seafood the best choice for omega-3s? As I mentioned on the previous page, DHA and EPA are the omega-3 fatty acids most directly involved in controlling fat metabolism. While the body can make its own DHA and EPA from ALA, the type of omega-3 found in plants, the conversion of ALA to DHA and EPA is inefficient. That's because the production of DHA and EPA requires vitamin B_6, magnesium, calcium, and zinc and is hindered by trans fats, cortisol, alcohol, and sugar. Therefore, while it certainly can't hurt to eat more ALA-rich foods (like walnuts, flaxseeds, flaxseed oil, and purslane), it's better to get most of your omega-3s from DHA- and EPA-rich foods, which happen to be primarily fish and seafood. (Note to vegetarians: The fish actually get their DHA and EPA from algae, so if you can find the algae, that would be a good vegetarian source of DHA and EPA. Since algae can be hard to find, in the meantime your best bet is to look for supplements made from algae.)

The best seafood sources of omega-3s are cold-water, oily fish, such as mackerel, herring, bluefish, salmon, and tuna. However, there are a host of contamination concerns surrounding today's seafood catch, specifically mercury and PCBs. In Chapter 9, I include a detailed section about how to buy and eat seafood safely.

If you don't eat fish, I recommend that you take a high quality fish oil in capsule or liquid form. Cod liver oil is the best fish oil supplement because it contains vitamins A and D along with omega-3 fats. Vitamin A helps you maintain healthy eyes, bones, teeth, and skin as well as benefits reproduction, prevents bladder stones, and acts as a cancer-preventing antioxidant. Vitamin D can prolong life; combat disease, infection, depression, pain, and inflammation; and give you stronger bones.

Yummy Real-Food Meals

Once you get into the swing of things, your day might start with an organic spinach omelet made from pasture-raised eggs with deep orange yolks, a bowl of sweet organic strawberries, and a glass of creamy whole raw or organic milk. Lunch could be a fragrant mixed greens salad tossed with olive oil and rich balsamic vinegar and topped with strips of naturally raised ham and quartered ripe heirloom tomatoes brought alive with a sprinkling of sea salt, followed by juicy organic watermelon chunks and cherries. Dinner might be a succulent lemon and rosemary roasted naturally raised chicken or slices of naturally raised roast beef; steamed organic asparagus sprinkled with herbes de Provence and drizzled with melted organic butter; crisp russet potato quarters roasted with coconut oil and seasoned with sweet paprika, sea salt, and freshly ground black pepper; and a wonderfully bitter watercress salad that requires just a pinch of pungent olive oil. Raw cheese and tart organic apples would make up dessert.

How delicious does that lineup sound! That's the beauty of a real-food weight loss plan—it's not about going hungry or depriving yourself of the foods you love. When you eat real food, you discover a whole new respect for food, and you'll experience the most delicious meals you've ever tasted. Eating a diet of real food is not a struggle. Once you learn the ropes and get your routine down, every meal will be a treat. One of the best perks: You'll be overcome with an amazing peace of mind because you'll be confident that you're supplying your body with all the nutrients it needs to run at its best. And when you provide your body with the right nutrients, it will automatically shrink to your ideal body weight. Eating a balanced diet of real food will result in a trim, attractive body as things begin to run more smoothly on a cellular level.

Now that you have a clear understanding of how you can lose weight eating a diet of real food, the rest of the book will give you all the day-to-day practical guidance you need to make the conversion from factory food to a real-food diet and apply the real-food philosophy to losing weight.

Real-Foodie Kath Younger: Sunday Prep-Time

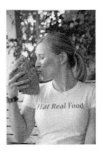

Out of college, Katherine Younger found herself about 30 pounds overweight and out of shape. That's when she decided to regain control of her health and weight and began her personal journey to a real-food diet. She began to educate herself about food, and as a result was able to make better food choices. In addition, she got moving and started exercising regularly. But Kath didn't do it alone; with the support of a private online community, she started sharing her struggles, her photos, and ultimately her success. Soon she had dropped 31 pounds.

Kath's transformation and her photographs of her meals were so inspiring that she was encouraged to move from the private online community to a blog. Thousands of readers now visit www.katheats.com each day, checking in on her posts. Along with the photographs, Kath includes stories about creating her meals, ingredient tips, and easy-to-follow recipes.

In January 2008, Kath embarked on a 3-year journey to return to school at Winthrop University in Rock Hill, South Carolina, to become a registered dietitian. She completed an internship through Winthrop in 2010 and became registered in August 2010. Now, in addition to writing, blogging, and building her career as an RD, she runs Great Harvest Bread Company, in Charlottesville, Virginia, with her husband. Visit Kath's blog often, and spend as much time as you can on it (you must read her fantastic article on oatmeal, which was also published in O *Magazine*)! Her recipes and outstanding photos will show you how truly gorgeous and joyful real food can be, and her advice on living a real-food lifestyle is beyond inspiring.

Kath finds experimenting with food adventurous and a delicious way to discover new favorite dishes. She says, "There's this mindset that food's either all 'fun and games' or 'all healthy' and no middle ground. But there is—it takes creativity to come up with healthy meals." Kath forgoes most processed foods and now uses simple, fresh ingredients. She's an advocate of keeping food diaries for those losing weight to track both what and how much you are consuming. Diaries are a way to gauge portions and to see how many of your calories are coming from the factory and how many from real foods.

Kath considers real food "food that our grandparents would have recognized. It's either grown from the ground or an animal naturally raised." However, that doesn't keep all prepackaged foods from Kath's meals. She notes some foods with simple ingredients that she adores, like dried fruit and nut bars, and that she may not have the time or the equipment to prepare. "Even though they come in a package, it's still real food on the inside that someone else has conveniently packaged for me."

Here are a few of Kath's tips for putting together a healthy meal.

- **Plan ahead:** "If you know you're not going to have time, cook when you do have the time so the prep work's been done."
- **Be creative:** How about pumpkin oatmeal pancakes? Or a green smoothie made with spinach?
- **Have a fully stocked refrigerator:** "You can't cook with what you don't have." Get a grocery list together and stick with it.

I asked Kath to take us through a Sunday prep day. It's the time she puts aside to make sure she has real food at the ready during the midweek crunch when life gets busy, busy, busy. Take it away, Kath!

Now that our weekdays have gotten much busier, I've gone back to my "Sunday prep day" ways just a bit.

Made nut butter
Made a giant pot of soup
Roasted beets!
Went grocery shopping

We should be all set for a busy week ahead! I always tell busy people the key to midweek healthy eating is just a wee bit of planning and chopping on Sundays. You can make a whole pot of stovetop oats to microwave during the week, chop all your veggies for salads, and even make lunches for the upcoming 5 days! I used to do it all when I had my stints of 8 a.m. to 9 p.m. classes straight through.

While the soup simmered, the beets roasted. This time I used regular beets—they are not NEARLY as good as the goldens, and they were much harder to peel!

Tonight's dinner was the Montana High Plains Wheat Berry Chili. Luckily I'm a pro at wheatberries. I simmered them, then added the spice pack and a 28-ounce can of tomatoes and some broth. The recipe called for ground turkey, but I used a can of kidney beans instead. No reason other than:

Organic turkey = $10
Beans = $1
Voilà, I had delicious chili topped with yogurt + cheese + tortilla chips!

Finally, do you know what one of my favorite desserts is? Making overnight oats and taking a bite before I put them in the fridge for breakfast! The sweet banana milk is the perfect one-bite dessert. ☺

CHAPTER 7

Real-Food Rehab

Throughout my years treating clients for weight loss, I've treated many folks with food addiction issues. But Molly was one of my more hardcore cases. Chocolate was Molly's addictive food of choice, and thanks to the factory food culture we live in, opportunities for her to succumb to her vice were endless. Godiva bars at the bookstore. Double chocolate chip cookies at the kiosk in the mall. Kit Kats in the vending machine at the office. Ben & Jerry's Chocolate Fudge Brownie ice cream at the 7-Eleven a block from her house. Raisinets at the movie theater (thrown into a tub of salty, buttery popcorn). Her favorite "fancy" dark chocolate bar at the grocery store checkout.

Molly confided to me that whenever she'd get ready to go to any of her chocolate spots, she'd get super excited. She said it was the same feeling you get when you're packing for a fun-filled vacation. Her heart would even start beating faster, she said. And she admitted that there were times when she would actually make up excuses to go to the mall, the bookstore, or the 7-Eleven just to get chocolate. Once she even went to see a movie she wasn't the least bit interested in just so she could eat her infamous Raisinets/popcorn combo. There were times, she said, when she felt out of control.

Molly certainly isn't alone in her experience with food addiction. In fact, the way our food culture is set up, with a candy counter, vending machine, and coffee shop at every corner, it's impossible in America to avoid the temptation of addictive food. The good news is that the scientific community is on it. And one of the main things they've figured out so far is that *just saying no* to the foods you're addicted to does not work. Period. Attempts to resist in that way will only end up increasing your cravings. What the body of research on this topic has concluded is that first and foremost, it's time to stop framing overeating as a lack of willpower, and start viewing it as a biological issue. When it comes to food addiction, haywire brain chemistry is often at the root of the problem.

So in order to gain control over food cravings, you must first accept that you're doing battle with your own brain, and that's a powerful adversary. Another important finding is that, once established, the connections in our brains that have formed a habit can never fully be cut. (A "habit" in this sense is when a certain behavior has reached a level where it is automatic. For instance, you come home from work and automatically walk to the cupboard and grab a bag of chips without even thinking about it.) But don't worry! The good news is, there are a number of tools you can use to *overcome* the behavior in the short term. In the long term, by adopting and repeating *new* behaviors, you can establish good habits that over time will become just as strong as the old ones. Once this happens, those old bad habits will cool down, recede into the background, and grow cobwebs. And just like any old, dusty relic in a hidden corner of your attic, it would take a heck of a lot to bring them out again.

Nonetheless, for the purposes of both ending your overeating habit and getting off factory food, it's important to understand that there will be a hump to get over. Because of this hump, which could last anywhere from a few weeks to even a few months, many people throw in the towel. Really understanding that you're up against a biological issue, and *not* a lack of willpower, helps you stay the course and not give up. It's also important to keep in mind that the hump I'm talking about is a period of time that is all about healing, and just like with any other physical and mental issue, the healing takes time and patience on your part. If you relapse, pull up your fabulous bootstraps and get right back on track. Don't pull the old, "Well, I fell off the wagon, now I can bury my face in chocolate or chips or Ho Hos and try again on Monday or the first of next month or next New Year's," routine. When you go that route, you're giving yourself permission to overeat and you're giving in to the whacked out chemical scramble in your brain. Instead, stop viewing the transgression as a full-on flop off the wagon, see it as just a very minor slip, and hop right back up and on track.

Those tools I mentioned above will help you stay the course. And they have science to back 'em up, so they work! My goal for this chapter is to provide you with an entire toolbox of strategies to help you get past the hump. Not every single tool will work for you. And one might not work for you one day, but on another day, it might be just the thing.

Rehab Toolbox

There's been tons of research done on overcoming addictive behaviors— from food addiction to drug addiction and cigarette addiction. Out of all that research, it turns out there are four main courses of action a person can take to succeed in overcoming their addictive behavior:

- Becoming aware

- Embracing competing behavior

- Thinking competing thoughts

- Finding support

BECOME AWARE

"Becoming aware" means that you need to sit down, maybe even with a pen and paper, and first figure out what the foods are you have issues with, and second, what the situations or "cues" are that lead you to eat them. So grab your Real-Food Notebook, and make a list of the foods on one page (or five pages, if that's what it takes). On another page, map out all of the cues that lead you down the path that ends with your eating an entire quart of ice cream, a supersize anything, or whatever your food of choice is.

What the research shows is that so-called "sensory signals," like driving past your favorite ice cream shop or smelling fried food cooking, can be cues to out-of-control eating. Other examples include driving past your favorite fast food restaurant; going to a coffeehouse at lunch with your co-worker; going to the movies, smelling the popcorn, and seeing all the candy behind the counter; and walking past the vending machine at the office. Stressful situations can also be cues. For instance, you may tend to get out of control with your eating when you're up against a tight deadline, you just sat in crazy traffic or had a negative confrontation, or you have to face something that makes you fearful or anxious, like public speaking or a job interview.

Why am I asking you to make these lists? These lists will give you all the info you need in order to know what you're up against. It might be that your eating is so out of control that you have never really sat down to make sense of which foods are your biggest weaknesses. Taking time to focus on this will organize your patterns and show you which foods you need to be vigilant about. What's more, the lists will help you understand what foods are going to be difficult for you to give up. Once you

When Good Habits Become Automatic

So how long will it take you to get over the hump? Do new good habits ever become as automatic as the old ones? The answer to the second question is yes. In fact, research shows this to be the case. Now, to answer the first question about how much time it takes, I defer to research recently published in the *European Journal of Social Psychology*. It was found that on average a new behavior—whether it was starting to exercise, or giving up a certain food—was adopted after 66 days. But remember that this is an average, so variations occur. The habits examined in the study took anywhere from 18 to 254 days to form. As you'd imagine, drinking a daily glass of water became automatic very quickly, but doing 50 sit-ups before breakfast required more dedication. The researchers also noted that missing a single day did not reduce the chance of forming a new good habit. So remember, if you slip, just get right back up.

become aware of your trouble zones, you can take steps to avoid them. Take a different route home from work, one that doesn't pass that wafting French fry smell. Or decline those coffee runs with your colleague, if a coffeehouse is your trigger. Or, easiest of all, don't stock your fridge and pantry with your danger foods. However, in our factory food world, it's not always going to be possible for you to bypass temptation. At those times, being aware of your food vices and the cues that cause you to eat them will allow you to "self-monitor." Before you give into a bad habit, you do have a few initial seconds to prevent yourself from succumbing. If you are in self-monitor mode, you are more likely to be alert enough to take advantage of those few seconds and put on the brakes. Okay, so what can you do in those few seconds to avoid overeating? Read on.

EMBRACE COMPETING BEHAVIOR

Embracing competing behavior is a tool you can implement after you've gained awareness of your cues. If you have that competing behavior at the ready, it can be one of the actions you take in those first few seconds in situations where you're tempted to succumb to the food you're working to get over. I call having a competing behavior at the ready "if-then planning." Here's an example of how if-then planning works: "If I begin to crave chocolate because I just walked past the vending machine at work, instead I will then go and grab the yummy yogurt snack I prepared for myself if a cue like this came up." Bam! Wacky Brain Chemicals: 0, You: 1!

Here's another example: "If someone asks me if I want a cupcake, I say 'No thank you, I'm off sugar for health reasons.' And then I grab my cute new to-go container (more on these below), which has a handful of my favorite raw unsalted nuts in it (I love me some raw, unsalted cashews—they are divine!) and I eat those to satisfy any food craving my friend's invitation might have dredged up." This is a great example because the cue involves what I call a "sugar pusher." You know who they are. You might have even been one yourself back in the day. This is your co-worker or neighbor who is always offering you a cupcake or a brownie or some other confection that she baked up. Of course she likes you, and that's the main reason she's pushing the sugar at you, but there's also a more sinister reason. If you indulge in the sugary confection or two or three, she feels better about her habit. I know this from experience, as I used to be a sugar pusher myself back in the marshmallowy Golden Graham treat days. Having a stock answer like "I'm off sugar for health reasons" should stop the sugar pusher from a repeat offense. At the very least, she won't push as hard.

If-then planning is awesome, and it works. Well more than 100 studies, on everything from diet and exercise to time management, have shown that deciding beforehand *when* and *where* you will take *specific* steps to overcome a behavior can double or triple your chances for pulling it off. As shown in the two examples above, when it comes to giving up a certain food, a great if-then plan is to be ready to replace your food vice with healthy real food. For instance, instead of eating chips during my break, I'll bring a container of delicious diced fresh strawberries or mango and papaya squares or cool, juicy watermelon cubes—whatever fruit is in season and that you love. In fact, involving real food in your if-then planning actually ends up involving a powerful ally in your battle with your brain. That ally is dopamine.

Wait, what? Didn't I say in Chapter 1 that dopamine is the enemy? The truth is, dopamine can be both evil and good. Recall that dopamine is your brain's pleasure chemical. Well, pleasure isn't necessarily a bad thing! On the contrary, pleasure is usually a good thing! The pleasure you get from being outside in the sunshine or chatting with your BFF on the phone or making out with someone—dopamine is involved in all of these. So why not exploit it to form good eating habits? Recall that you can form good habits to replace the bad ones. The way to go about it is to make eating real, healthy food as enjoyable as possible. When you make eating real food an enjoyable, taste-filled experience, you will want to do it again and again. In fact, new pathways will be laid down in your brain. And instead of craving the foods that you want to stop eating, you'll begin craving healthy real foods.

To create that enjoyable, delicious experience, make the food delicious (just check out any of the recipes in the back of this book) and make the time you spend eating it special by serving it on dishes you love in a beautiful presentation. When I decided to make the switch from factory food to real food, one of the things I did was buy a few new pretty dishes to serve it on. This might sound silly, but hear me out. I love to cook, and like most folks who love to cook, I am a sucker for a pretty plate or an elegant bowl or a fabulous mug. You eat first with your eyes, and to me, presentation is an important aspect of savoring and enjoying your food. I also purchased a few cute, fun to-go containers. It was like buying a new outfit for a party you're looking forward to—the purchase enhances the experience.

So in the afternoon when I was jonesing for a snack, I'd cut up some gorgeous fresh strawberries and rinse off a handful of pretty ripe blueberries and then maybe add a thin slice of delicious, fresh-from-the-bakery whole grain bread, and I'd arrange it beautifully on one of my pretty new plates. I also bought myself a delightful food tray at the flea market (I think it cost me $4) on which to serve myself my afternoon snack. Sitting down to eat this elegant and delicious snack was such a treat. I felt like a grand lady. It made me happy. Overall, it was just a fun, satisfying experience. So the next time I was craving a snack, I craved strawberries and blueberries instead of gaudy, too-salty potato chips.

The great thing is that once you get over the hump, you won't have to go through so much effort to make eating real food a dopamine rush because you'll be back in your right mind, and you'll truly get how incredibly sexy, gorgeous, delicious, and satisfying real food is!

THINK COMPETING THOUGHTS

Taking action with if-then planning is not the only way to overcome a craving when you're cued. Another tool you can use involves changing the dialogue in your head. I call this "flipping your script." Here's how it works. When I would look at or think about Cheetos or Cheerios or any food I was trying to get off of, I would say to myself, "That's not going to make me feel good. That's disgusting. It's not real food. It won't satisfy me, I'd rather have something that will make me feel good."

Flipping the script in my head allowed me to take the power from the food just by changing how I perceived it. And everything I said in my new script echoed what I felt, so it had real power. After repeating your new script over and over again, in time it becomes second nature, and anytime you begin to think of going for the foods you're trying to avoid, you'll automatically talk yourself back to reality, and you'll be way less likely to go after them. Take some time as you begin your journey to formulate your own personal script in your head, or write it down if you like. If a certain food makes you feel tired and lethargic after you eat it, adding that detail can also be powerful because you'll recall that sick feeling, and that negative twinge of memory will help you to avoid the food all the more.

Mighty Motivation

There is always some kind of motivating factor behind anyone's decision to turn over a new leaf. Another great tool for getting over the hump is to keep near you during those first few months a physical reminder of whatever your motivation is. For instance, if your motivation is to physically feel better, you might cut out a photo from a magazine of someone about your age who is engaged in a healthy activity or who just looks all-around healthy. Tape it to places you see during your daily routine, like the edge of your computer screen, your bathroom mirror, your fridge, or the cover of your daily planner. If you have kids, you might be motivated to be fit and healthy so you can be there for them as long as possible or be a good role model for them. Keeping photos of your children in these same spots may remind you of this.

Another idea is to make what I call a "dream board, " also known as a motivation board. Give your dream board a place of prominence in your home. I have personally been doing this for years and I firmly believe that it has played a significant role in helping my dreams turn into realities. To do this, simply buy a bulletin board or even a large piece of poster board, whatever works for you, and attach inspiring photos, magazine clippings, and quotations to it. Be creative with it. Don't bring any negativity to your motivational dream board. Always keep the message positive. You will be surprised at how much having a physical reminder of your motivations for adopting a healthier lifestyle will help you to stay on track.

FIND SUPPORT

The final tool is so important I've devoted all of Chapter 10 to it: real-food community support. I firmly believe that when it comes to switching off bad eating habits and switching on good ones, having a community that can support you is vital, and this is especially true for making the switch to real food. In Chapter 10, I introduce you to many amazing real-food pioneers who offer you the most incredible guidance and support. They are super-cool people. They're not about judging you or making you feel out of the loop. They're funny, smart, down-to-earth folks on their own unique journeys, and they're willing to share the deets with you to help and support you (and to help themselves—who knows, maybe there's a real-food blogger waiting to come out in you!). Plus, there are the real-food gurus, like Mark Bittman, who are at the forefront of the movement and are so fantastic to learn from. Not to mention organizations, meetups, swaps, and more. It's a vibrant, fantastic, growing community of support, and it's just waiting to welcome you with open arms. Chapter 10 is devoted to showing you exactly how you can become a card-carrying member of the real-food community.

There's another level of support you're going to need as you start your journey, and that's the support of your family and friends. My hope for you is that the people in your life will support you, and even help you as you start out, whether they are also on the real-food track or not. But don't expect everyone in your life to be supportive. Eating is personal, and it's highly ingrained in our sense of who we are. It is a super-emotional issue for a lot of people. So be prepared, and if someone in your life is less than supportive, just remind yourself that it's your health and happiness on the line and that the stakes are too high to be swayed by someone else's lack of understanding. On the other side, if there are some real-foodies in your life—your sister, BFF, or co-worker—reach out to them and have a conversation about what they're doing and what advice they have to share. Take my word for it, they'll be thrilled to chat with you about real food; it's something folks get excited about. The great thing is that enthusiasm is contagious!

Dr. Amy Reichenbach: What to Do When Food Addiction Becomes Emotional

Working at Passages Malibu has given me a great deal of insight into the struggle against addiction. In addition, my experience there has allowed me access to some amazing experts on the topic. One of those experts is clinical psychologist Dr. Amy Reichenbach. She has treated many people with food addictions, and I asked her to give me her take on the emotional issues at play when someone develops addictive issues with food. Here's how she approaches the issue of emotional eating.

Most individuals are not overweight because they want to be; they have unknowingly become addicted to certain types of food. Food addiction is not something that is consciously chosen, but rather a dependency that is caused by both physiological and psychological factors. Nonetheless, most food addicts feel deep shame about their eating and food choices. They confuse their unhealthy eating habits for a lack of willpower or a sign of internal weakness. Food addiction actually has nothing to do with weakness, gluttony, or indulgence. This by no means suggests that you are powerless over food. In fact it's the opposite; once you arm yourself with this knowledge you will finally be empowered with the necessary tools to take control of your eating and health.

The Biological Component

New scientific research shows that our brains and bodies often become physically addicted to factory foods. In fact, sugar seems to stimulate the brain's reward centers with the neurotransmitter dopamine exactly like other addictive drugs do. In short, research is showing that we may need to literally "detox" off factory foods the same way we would addictive drugs.

The Psychological Component

In conjunction with this physical addiction, our minds become psychologically addicted to unhealthy eating behaviors. Psychological addiction differs from physical addiction in that even after the body is restored to a healthy state of physical functioning, the mind continues to remember and crave the emotional reward. In other words, even after being fully detoxed from factory foods, we may return to these foods for emotional reasons. This explains why many individuals relapse back into food addiction even long after their hormones and neurochemicals have been returned to a state of balance.

Psychological addiction is most often caused by unresolved emotional issues that lay below our level of awareness in the subconscious. They can be responsible for unhealthy food choices and ultimately the vicious cycle of food addiction. This means we are not eating out of physical hunger or to wisely nourish our bodies, but instead to relieve negative emotions or distract ourselves from repressed psychological distress.

Psychologically, high-calorie foods are often associated with good times or pleasant feelings. Most people have many happy experiences and memories involving food: holiday gatherings, romantic candlelit dinners, birthday celebrations, baking cookies with grandma, and pizza parties, just to name a few. Our senses are closely connected to our emotions, and the taste of a "comfort food" can emotionally bring us back to a more pleasant time almost immediately. Also, finding comfort or distraction in food may be a learned behavior. You may have been taught at an early age that food can comfort and distract from unpleasant feelings. Whatever the reason, our subconscious mind has learned that painful memories, thoughts, and feelings can be temporarily numbed or escaped by eating certain foods.

The Good News

The good news is we can reclaim the power from our subconscious and uncover these hidden feelings, bringing them to the light of day. This can be done by practicing mindfulness, journaling, and self-exploration. As these repressed feelings and thoughts begin to rise to the surface of our awareness it will be uncomfortable as we may initially experience anxiety, fear, anger, or depression. However, once we become aware of these issues we can confront, process, and resolve them. Then, our subconscious will no longer need to seek out food as a means of soothing or numbing repressed emotional pain. When your repressed feelings become conscious, you gain power and can finally start making the decisions you want.

To review, here are the steps toward curing food addiction from psychologist Dr. Amy Reichenbach's perspective.

1. Many of us are misinformed about what healthy eating is, so it's important to follow guidance, such as that offered in this book, to gain an understanding of exactly what it means to "eat healthfully."

2. Once the physical addiction is broken, and you are detoxified from factory foods (the hump described above), begin to explore the possibility of contributing psychological factors.

3. Examine your own thoughts, feelings, and memories in an accepting, nonjudgmental, and curious manner.

4. Journal about possible unresolved issues and repressed emotions. Do this in a stream-of-consciousness format, free of grammatical or spelling restraints. Pulling these repressed emotions to the forefront is the way for you to take charge over your subconscious, and once you are in the driver's seat, anything is possible.

5. If you find you're having difficulty analyzing your own thoughts and feelings, psychotherapy from a trained and licensed professional may be helpful.

Now that we've discussed at length the various tools you can deploy against cues while you're getting past the hump, let's review the contents of your toolbox:

- Become aware of the cues that cause you to eat the foods you want to avoid. Once you've gained this awareness, avoid those cues and/or self-monitor.

- Utilize "if-then planning": Have an action you're ready to take if faced with a cue. Remember, a great if-then plan is to substitute the factory food or food vice with real food.

- Make eating real food a dopamine-filled experience.

- Flip your script by changing your perception of what factory food is and what it does to you.

- Find support among real-foodies you know or within the real-food community (more on this in Chapter 10).

CHAPTER 8

Reality Bites, Or What Are You *Really* Eating?

People lie about what they eat. Research shows they claim to eat way less than they really do. Some studies show folks underreport their caloric intake by as much as 30 percent or more. On the other hand, when it comes to veggies, people lie in the other direction—insisting they eat far more than they actually do. We know we are expected to eat 5 or more servings of fruits and vegetables a day, so that's the amount most claim to eat. What's disturbing about this tendency to bend, twist, or disregard the truth is that more often than not, people actually believe their fabrications. So, at the end of the day, many folks are lying to *themselves* about what they're eating and in what amounts.

Before moving onto the next part of the book, I want you to make sure you're not living in your own food fantasyland. To empower you to come clean about your cuisine, instead of asking you to write down what you eat over a certain period of time in a food journal, I ask that you keep a food *photo journal* instead. Seeing is believing. In addition, with the help of the questions below, I ask that you analyze what you're eating. For a dash of added guidance, I've provided a sample food photo journal from a friend of mine who agreed to play guinea pig, along with a complete analysis of her meals and an alternative menu plan for her. Finally, this chapter concludes with a section that takes the question "what are you *really* eating?" to the next level by giving you the dirt on exactly what you're consuming when you eat factory foods that contain ingredients that you can't even pronounce. Okay, get ready for your close-ups!

Food Photo Journaling

In order to come to grips with your current eating habits, for one week, take a photo of anything and everything you eat and drink before putting it into your mouth. Thanks to cell phone cameras and digital cameras, getting the shots shouldn't be all that difficult. At the end of the week, transfer the photos to your computer or iPad, whatever works best for you. Save them either in a special file on your computer titled "Photo Food Journal" or on a free Web site, like www.kodakgallery.com or www.snapfish.com—anywhere that will allow you to view the week's worth of food intake in an organized fashion. Next, pull out your trusty Real-Food Notebook and answer the following questions based on what you see in the photos. Check out the sample food photo journal in the following section to get some guidance on answering the questions and then provide your own overall analysis of your eating habits.

- How much of your diet for the week was processed factory food?

- How much would you consider to be real food?

- How many servings of fruits and/or veggies did you eat per day? Were there any days when you ate 5 servings (the USDA-recommended amount, and the minimum amount I recommend—more is better)?

- What percentage of your daily food intake do you estimate came from refined carbs?

- What kinds of fats are you eating? What proportion are real fats and what proportion factory fats? Did you eat any trans fats? (Hint: If the label says "partially hydrogenated vegetable oil," "hydrogenated oil," "vegetable shortening," "shortening," or "margarine," it's a trans fat.) If you're not sure, remember that if it's a processed food, chances are it contains either trans fat or polyunsaturated fats made from vegetables, seeds, or grains—the factory fats discussed in Chapter 4.

- Is there a particular food that is a weakness for you? Does that food cause you to overeat in a food-addicted kind of way?

- Did you feel out of sorts or have a stomachache after eating any of your meals or snacks? If so, which foods were the culprits?

- List the foods you ate that were a good source of natural fiber (as opposed to added synthetic fiber, like that found in many sugary cereals).

- List any foods you ate that were a good source of omega-3 fatty acids.

Julie's Food Photo Journal

I asked a friend of mine, Julie, to keep a 2-day journal of everything she ate and drank (besides water), including a photo of each food she recorded. Take a look at her responses to the questions and my analysis of her eating habits. Finally, check out the alternative 2-day real-food menu I devised for her.

JULIE'S ANALYSIS

How much of your diet for those 2 days consisted of processed factory food?

I would say that roughly more than 80 percent of what I ate those 2 days was processed factory food. Plus, a couple of the meals that weren't primarily processed factory foods, like the tacos and the sloppy joe, also had components in them that came from the food factory, like the white sesame bun and the taco shells.

How much would you say was real food?

I would say that around 15 percent or possibly less could be considered real food. I suppose the fixin's in the taco shells, the sloppy joe meat and the salads on the side of the sloppy joe meal, plus the Chinese takeout, could be considered real food.

How many servings of fruits and veggies did you eat per day? Were there any days when you ate 5 servings?

Most likely, you could eke out one serving of fruits and veggies each day. On day one, the tomatoes and lettuce in the tacos and the bell peppers on the pizza together are probably one serving of veggies. And on day two, the lettuce and other veggies in the salad and the few veggies in the Chinese lo mien and fried rice are likely at least one serving of veggies. No, there wasn't a day where I ate 5 servings of fruits and veggies.

How many of the foods you ate contained refined carbs? (Just give an estimate. For instance, you could count the number of meal, snack, and beverage photos that contain an item with refined carbs, then divide by the total number of photos in your diary—these aren't scientific measurements I'm asking for, just good guestimates.)

Out of the 13 photos I took, which included my meals and snacks, nine had foods that contain refined sugar, turns out even the yogurt, which I thought was healthy, was extremely high in sugar when I thought it was a good protein source . . . who knew! I'm no good at math, but according to my handy dandy calculator, about 70 percent of my meals and snacks had some form or another of refined carbs in them.

What kinds of fats did you eat? What proportion were real fats and what proportion factory fats? Did you eat any trans fats? (Hint: If the label says "partially hydrogenated vegetable oil," "hydrogenated oil," "vegetable shortening," "shortening," or "margarine," it's a trans fat. If you're not sure, remember that if it's a processed food, chances are it has trans fat. Just take a guess.

In pretty much every meal and snack I ate, some form of fat was involved, which, after reading the chapter on fats in this book, I now know is not a bad thing. I now get that it's the type of fat that matters. Unfortunately, it seems most of the fats in the foods I ate were the "bad" kind. Many of the foods I ate had trans fats in them; from the donut, which was fried in partially hydrogenated soybean oil, to the Baked! Cheetos to the frozen pizza. And when I wasn't eating trans fat, it seems I was eating the other kind of factory fat, polyunsaturated vegetable oils, like soy oil in the Nutri-Grain bar I ate—even the Planters Mixed Nuts had POs! As for the saturated fat that was in the ground meat I ate in my sloppy joe and my tacos, I'm not sure, but I'm betting it wasn't from grass fed cows, so I'm assuming it was also high in omega-6 fats since the cows were likely fed some kind of grain. I'm not sure, but I don't think any healthy "real" fats slipped into my food in those 2 days. Boo!

Is there a particular food that is a weakness for you? Does that food cause you to overeat in a food-addicted kind of way?

For me, my downfall is salty foods. For instance, after I made the extra effort to eat the Baked! Cheetos, I was still hungry and got a bag of buttered popcorn! The next night, my intention was just to eat a handful of the mixed nuts, but after eating one, I just kept eating another and another and another, and pretty soon the tin was empty.

Did you feel out of sorts or have a stomachache after eating any of your meals or snacks? If so, which foods were the culprits?

To be honest, about a year ago, I developed what my doctor says is acid reflux. So these days I always have an out-of-sorts stomach.

List the foods you ate that were a good source of natural fiber (as opposed to added synthetic fiber, like that found in many sugary cereals).

I would say that the only food I ate that was a good source of natural fiber were the nuts, but they contained a good deal of salt and added oil. I had assumed that the Nutri-Grain bar was high in fiber, but after reading the ingredients label, I'm thinking the high-fructose corn syrup, other refined carbs, and various additives and preservatives disqualify it from being a "healthy" source of fiber.

List any foods you ate that were a good source of omega-3 fatty acids.

None of the foods I ate were a good source of omega-3 fatty acids.

MY ANALYSIS

After having Julie answer the Food Photo Journal questions, I wanted to analyze her eating habits myself to help give you a sense of where I'm going with the questions I asked you to answer, and to help you analyze your own eating habits.

The first thing that struck me after looking over Julie's journal was the high amount of refined carbs she is eating and drinking. Nearly every meal and snack contained some form of refined carb, either in the form of high-fructose corn syrup or refined flour. After reading Chapters 1 and 3, you now get how harmful a diet high in unrefined carbs can be. It plays a role in a myriad of terrible health problems, like type 1 diabetes and heart disease, plus it makes us eat too much. The amount of unrefined carbs she eats plays a role in Julie's overeating. From the photos, it looks like Julie's portions are out of control. Five tacos and an entire plate of side "salads" with her sloppy joe—these portion sizes are way too big. Plus, she's snacking way too much between meals—the chips, the candy bar, the fritter. All that snacking tells me that she's eating to fill the hysterical hunger caused by unstable blood sugar, which is the result of eating too many refined carbs.

The second thing I noticed is that not only is she eating too many fatty foods, the fats she's eating are nearly all unhealthy factory fats. Even the nuts, which are high in natural fats, had partially hydrogenated oil added to them. Another factory fat she's getting is trans fats, perhaps the worst food ingredient out there. Trans fats are e-v-i-l; not only do they raise total cholesterol levels, they also deplete good cholesterol (HDL), which helps protect against heart disease. If that wasn't bad enough, she's also eating way too much polyunsaturated fat (PO) from factory-processed vegetable oils. These are not cool for two reasons: one, eating too much of them contributes to a vast imbalance in Julie's omega-6 to omega-3 ratio. As discussed in Chapter 4, we ideally need an omega-6 to omega-3 ratio of 2 to 1. From the looks of it, Julie got loads of omega-6 fats and no omega-3 fats, which could lead her to have a higher risk of heart disease and even certain cancers. While one source of omega-3s is meat from grass fed animals, I doubt the meat from her sloppy joe and tacos was from grass fed cows. The second reason eating foods high in POs is bad for you is that many experts believe the processing of the oil could be linked to cancer and heart disease.

The third thing I noticed is that because Julie's diet is so high in processed factory foods, it's full of potentially harmful additives and preservatives. In fact, nearly every processed food Julie ate contained at least one of the most dangerous food additives out there. (For more on exactly why these additives are dangerous, see Food Additives: Mystery Ingredients on page 98.) For instance, the sodas contain caramel color, and other food items on her list contain TBHQ (an antioxidant that comes from petroleum and is related to butane), food dyes, MSG, sodium nitrate, BHA, and BHT, all of which are on my "run, don't walk!" list of food additives.

Moreover, even if the additives in the foods Julie is eating aren't necessarily the most dangerous ones out of the thousands used by the factory food industry, it's fair to say she's ingesting an awful lot of stuff she is not even aware of. Take the carmine in the yogurt she ate; it's made from dried, ground-up red beetles. Look for this coloring in, among other foods, yogurt, candy, and juice drinks (pass the beetle juice!). It's actually harmless for most people, but there's certainly a huge "ick" factor, and vegetarians in particular might want to know about it. On top of these additives, Julie's many processed food choices, as well as her choices to eat out and order in, all caused her to consume copious amounts of added salt.

Finally, I'm concerned about what Julie is *not* eating. She's missing out on all the vitamins, minerals, and fiber in yummy fruits and veggies. Speaking of fiber, she's hardly getting any, as is also the case with omega-3s. So while she's eating high amounts of refined carbs, factory fats, salt, and a slew of food additives, she's getting hardly any of the nutrients her body needs to function properly.

Now that Julie has a better sense of what she's really eating as well as what she's missing out on, I'm excited to give her some real food alternatives. Below is a menu of 2 days' worth of real foods.

DAY ONE

Breakfast: Greek yogurt with raspberries and a handful of almond slivers

Hot green tea with a scoop of delicious cold-pressed coconut oil

Snack: Gorgeous grapes or sliced apples, papaya, pineapple, strawberries, or whatever fruit is in season accompanied by some amazing raw almonds, sliced and beautifully arranged in a lovely bowl or small plate, or carried to work with you in your favorite to-go container.

Lunch: Three fish tacos, small lettuce and tomato side salad.

Dinner: Grilled Margarita Pizza (page 242)

Fresh heirloom tomato salad

Breakfast: Lemony Blueberry Muffins (see page 195) with two hard-cooked free range eggs

Snack: A handful of unsalted cashews and an orange

Lunch: Farmers' Market "Tortilla" Soup (see page 213)

Dinner: Citrus Salmon with Asian Quinoa Salad (see page 222)

Or, if you'd like to pick up some "real" fast food, check out Chipotle if there's one in your area and get a burrito bowl with chicken, beans, and lots of veggies.

Food Additives: Mystery Ingredients

In the spirit of showing you what you're really eating, I'd like to spend some time discussing food additives. For so long we've taken it for granted that our food products contain mystery ingredients that we can't spell or pronounce, and that we have only the foggiest knowledge about. Take a moment to think about just how crazy this is: If someone walked up to you with a bowl that contained a strange looking powder, paste, or liquid, gave you a spoon, and said, "Dig in!" would you? Of course you wouldn't. But, in effect, that's what you're doing every single time you

Did You Know . . .

The U.S. Food and Drug Administration (FDA) has a list of food additives "generally recognized as safe," or "GRAS," many of which *have not undergone any testing.* The list, which contains approximately 700 items, is evaluated on an ongoing basis. A "safe" additive is defined by Congress as one about which there is "reasonable certainty that no harm will result from use." Some substances that are found to be harmful to people or animals may be allowed, but only at the level of 1/100th of the amount that is considered harmful. Additives on the GRAS list (that therefore may be found in your food) include methylparaben, which is known to have some endocrine-disrupting effects, and propyl gallate, which some experts link to cancer.

eat a factory food item that contains an ingredient you're clueless about. In the U.S., more than 3,000 substances can be added to foods for the purposes of preservation, coloring, texture, flavor, and more. It's this stuff that makes a 100-calorie cup of yogurt taste like key lime pie or enables a cream-filled cake to remain edible for decades.

What's the big deal about food additives? Many of them are poorly tested and possibly dangerous. Again, think about what that *really* means. It means that a substance that might come from, say, tar or petroleum or some other matter that humans are not designed to ingest is added to your food without rigorous testing that would ensure it's not going to harm you in any way.

"Run, Don't Walk!" Additives

While some food additives may indeed turn out to be perfectly safe for human consumption, there is a growing list of food additives that have been under scrutiny for their potentially harmful effects. All of these additives are on my "run, don't walk!" list. If you see any one of them on an ingredient label, take a pass.

Acesulfame-K. An artificial sweetener about 200 times sweeter than sugar that's found in baked goods, chewing gum, gelatin desserts, and soft drinks. Two rat studies have found that this substance may cause cancer; no other studies to prove this additive's safety have been conducted.

Artificial Coloring. An FDA study released in the spring of 2011 found that kids with ADHD may have a "unique intolerance" to artificial food colorings, suggesting there may be some truth in the common wisdom that synthetic food dyes make children more hyper. In addition, some dyes have been linked to adrenal gland, kidney, or brain tumors, or may contain some cancer-causing agents. The dyes in the study, which give bright color to beverages, cakes, pies, cereals, candies, and snack foods, are FD&C Blue 1 and 2; FD&C Green 3, Orange B, FD&C Red 3, FD&C Red 40, and FD&C Yellow 5 and 6. Also steer clear of Citrus Red 2 and Violet 1; their safety is not fully proven because of inconclusive data.

BHA and BHT. Butylated hydroxyanisole and butylated hydroxytoluene are used to keep fats and oils from going rancid. Commonly found in cereals, chewing gum, vegetable oil, and potato chips (and also in some food packaging to preserve freshness), these additives have been found in some studies to cause cancer in rats.

Caramel Coloring. Federal regulations describe four types of caramel coloring. All of them start out with some form of sugar. One is called "plain caramel." A second involves reacting sugar with sulfites. Another is made by reacting sugars with ammonium compounds. And in the fourth variety, the kind used in Coke and Pepsi, sugars are reacted with both ammonium and sulfite compounds. Reacting sugars with ammonia results in the formation of numerous chemical byproducts, two of which have been shown in government studies to promote lung, liver, and thyroid tumors in laboratory rats and mice. Since no distinction is made between the four types of caramel coloring on labels, you're better off avoiding them all.

Monosodium Glutamate (MSG). MSG is used as a flavor enhancer in many packaged foods, including soups, salad dressings, sausages, hot dogs, canned tuna, potato chips, and many more. MSG is a neurotoxic substance that causes many adverse reactions in sensitive individuals such as dizziness, violent diarrhea, and even anaphylactic shock. Longer term and more insidious consequences of MSG ingestion include Parkinson's and Alzheimer's in adults and neurological damage in children. Animal studies have linked MSG with brain lesions, retinal degeneration, and obesity. The factory food industry has figured out a way to disguise it on labels, so don't think you're safe just because you don't see "MSG" on the ingredient list. (See Chapter 9 for the complete lowdown.) For example, if an ingredient list says "flavoring," "seasoning," or "spices," there's probably MSG in the food. Another alias for MSG is "yeast extract." I have actually spotted "yeast extract" in supposedly "all-natural, organic" snack foods at health food stores, most of which were marketed to kids, so be on the lookout!

Olestra. Olestra is a fat substitute used in crackers and potato chips and marketed under the brand name Olean. This synthetic fat is not absorbed by the body (instead it goes right through), so it can cause diarrhea, loose stools, abdominal cramps, and flatulence, along with other effects. Furthermore, olestra reduces the body's ability to absorb benefi-cial fat-soluble nutrients, including lycopene, lutein, and beta-carotene.

Potassium Bromate. This additive is used in breads and rolls to increase the volume and as a texturizer. Although most bromate breaks down into bromide, which is harmless, the bromate that does remain causes cancer in animals. Bromate has been banned everywhere in the world except for the U.S. and Japan.

Propyl Gallate. This preservative, used to prevent fats and oils from spoiling, might cause cancer. It's used in vegetable oil, meat products, potato sticks, chicken soup base, and chewing gum, and is often used with BHA and BHT.

Saccharin. An artificial sweetener often found in "diet," "no-sugar-added" factory foods, soft drinks, and sweetener packets. Many studies on animals have shown that saccharin can cause various cancers. Other studies have shown that saccharin increases the potency of other cancer-causing chemicals. And the best epidemiology study (done by the National Cancer Institute) found that the use of artificial sweeteners (saccharin and cyclamate) was associated with a higher incidence of bladder cancer.

Sodium Nitrate. Sodium nitrite (or sodium nitrate) is used as a pre-servative, coloring, and flavoring in bacon, ham, hot dogs, luncheon meats, corned beef, smoked fish, and other processed meats. These additives can lead to the formation of cancer-causing chemicals called nitrosamines. Some studies have found a link between the consump-tion of cured meats and cancer in humans.

TBHQ. Tertiary butylhydroquinone comes from petroleum and is related to butane. It is often used as a preservative, applied either to the carton of fast food items or sprayed directly onto foods. Consuming just 5 grams of TBHG can be fatal. It's found in such trace amounts that it's highly unlikely you could eat that much at one time (it would take 312.5 chicken nuggets to consume a single gram of TBHQ), but still be wary.

Okay Additives

The previous list is the worst of the worst, but not all additives are as scary as BHT and MSG. Some, like guar gum and lecithin, are actually acceptable. Let's take a closer look at some of these additives.

Amylase is an enzyme that occurs naturally in plants, saliva, pancreatic juice, and microorganisms. Bakers add amylase to bread dough to serve as food for the fermenting yeast and also for better tasting, better toasting bread. Amylase also improves the dough's consistency and the bread's shelf life.

Guar gum is naturally sourced and originates from the seeds of guar beans. After guar beans are husked, milled, and screened, you're left with just guar endosperm, which is nutritious material surrounding the embryo. Grind that endosperm up and you're left with a fine powder. In foods, guar gum is used as a thickening agent—an emulsifier that prevents the separation of oil and water. You'll find guar gum on the ingredient label of many dairy products, particularly ice cream, where it works to maintain that smooth, soft texture. It's also in some baked goods and dressings.

Lecithin is found in animal and plant tissues such as egg yolk and soybeans. It's added to foods like chocolate, baked goods, and ice cream to keep oil and water from separating, to retard rancidity, and to make cakes fluffier.

Sorbic acid occurs naturally in many plants. A safe additive, it's found in cheese, syrup, jelly, wine, and dry fruits, and is added to prevent the growth of mold.

Xanthan gum is another natural food additive commonly found in sauces and dressings. Your favorite bottled barbecue sauce probably owes its perfect texture to xanthan gum, and usually a small amount will do the trick. Some gluten free baked goods use xanthan gum to add volume, so you'll find it at most health foods stores. Xanthan gum gets its name from *Xanthomonas campestris*, a bacteria. To make the additive, some form of sugar is fermented with the bacteria, typically corn syrup or a derivative of corn syrup.

I hope this chapter helps you gain acceptance of what it is you're really eating, because I believe it's an important step in making the journey from a factory food diet to a real-food diet. On top of that, if you want to lose weight, it's super important for you to be completely realistic and honest about what and how much you're eating. Now, it's time to take the next step—putting everything we've talked about into practice! Let's go get real!

PART III

Real Food in the Real World

CHAPTER 9

Supermarket
Survival Guide

By this point, you are armed with the information you need to understand what's real food and fake food and everything in between. But having the information is one thing; actually going out into the world and putting it into practice is a whole 'nother ball game. This final section of the book is meant to give you the guidance you need to go out into our factory food world and gather real food. In a way, we've come full circle. Our earliest ancestors had to gather, forage, and even experiment to find nutrients in their uncertain environment, and that's similar to the adventure you're embarking on. Take heart. Our ancestors found some pretty amazing foods on their search, and so will you! Our first stop is the supermarket.

As Michael Pollan notes, "A lot of food in a supermarket is not really food, but an edible food-like substance." But there is real food to be had there. In this chapter, to help you find the real food and avoid the factory food, I take you through the supermarket section by section and show you how to shop for real foods. You'll learn to navigate the treacherous inner shelves that are loaded with processed foods by becoming a bona fide label detective. In addition, I'll take you through the dairy, meat, seafood, and produce departments. Plus, you'll learn why diet foods make us fat, how to shop for real food at budget stores like Costco, Walmart, and Trader Joe's, and much, much more! Grab your basket and let's go!

The Inner Aisles: Become a Label Detective

The inner aisles of the supermarket are where the majority of factory foods are stocked. But because the food industry is tuned into the consumer demand for healthier, more natural food, they've begun using terminology in their marketing to make their heavily processed food items sound healthier than they are. For instance, some sugary cereals are now being hawked as "a great way to keep kids healthy," thanks to the fact that they have fiber. What the marketing doesn't point out is that the "fiber" is synthetic and doesn't do the same thing in our bodies as natural fiber. Not to mention the fact that these cereals contain heaping amounts of trans fat, artificial colorings, and preservatives. Or that, as you learned in Part I, the technology used to turn grain into colorful little O's renders its protein toxic.

And don't lull yourself into a false sense of security if you're shopping at a natural food supermarket. Deep-fried, heavily salted potato chips as well as candy, cookies, and other various boxed, bagged, canned, and shrink-wrapped foods sold at natural food supermarket chains are likely to be just as bad for you as those sold at regular supermarkets. So when you get to the inner aisles of the supermarket, whether it's a natural food chain, a regular supermarket chain, or a small, family-owned

---

Eat Real Food Instead of Fake Food

Granola or oatmeal instead of cereal
Olive oil and vinegar instead of bottled salad dressing
Coconut oil instead of vegetable oil

---

supermarket, at the end of the day, it's all about the ingredients listed on the labels. In order to navigate the trickery and confusion, you have to be ready to do a bit of detective work. In this section, my goal is to turn you into a full-on label detective.

Keep an Eye out for Misleading or False Label Lingo

Although food labels are supposed to tell us exactly what's in the food we're buying, marketers have created a language all their own to make foods sound more healthful than they really are. While some of those label claims are regulated by the FDA or monitored by the industry, and actually mean something, most health related claims, like "all natural," "doctor recommended," and "reduced fat," are misleading or false. The bottom line is that front-of-package labeling is about marketing, not health. At its worst, it misleads us into thinking food that is bad for us is healthful.

Below are several common but misleading claims.

- **"Lightly sweetened" or "low sugar":** The FDA has regulations concerning the use of "sugar free" and "no added sugars," but nothing governing the claims "low sugar" or "lightly sweetened." Be aware that the factory food industry will often include a number of different kinds of sugar in the ingredients list so it doesn't seem there is an excessive amount of any one kind of sugar, and it spaces them out, putting other ingredients in between to throw you farther off the trail. Below is a complete list of possible added sugars. If you see any one of them in an ingredient list, it's not the end of the world; however, if you see multiple added sugars, don't buy it—case closed!

  - *Added sugars*: Agave nectar; corn sweetener; corn syrup or corn syrup solids; dehydrated cane juice; dextrin; dextrose; fructose; fruit juice concentrate; glucose; high-fructose corn syrup; honey; invert sugar; lactose; maltodextrin; malt syrup; maltose, maple syrup; molasses; raw sugar; rice syrup; saccharose; sorghum; sucrose; syrup; treacle; turbinado sugar; xylose.

- **"A good source of fiber":** More often than not, this "fiber" doesn't come from traditional sources like whole grains, beans, vegetables, or fruit. Instead, the food industry is adding something called "isolated fibers" made from chicory root or purified powders of polydextrose and other substances into the product, all of which *have not* been shown to lower blood sugar or cholesterol.

- **"Strengthens your immune system":** Through crafty wording, food companies can get around FDA rules and give consumers the impression that a food item will ward off disease. If you see this claim on a food item, it's more than likely just an empty promise.

- **"Made with real fruit":** Often the "real fruit" is found in small quantities and isn't even the same kind of fruit pictured on the package.

- **"Made with whole grains":** Back in 2005, the FDA recommended consuming whole grains. Since then, a barrage of companies have given lip service to that advice by adding tiny doses of whole grains to their products. For instance, I picked up a loaf of bread that claimed to be "made with whole grains" on its packaging, and the first ingredient was enriched wheat flour, which is just ordinary, nutrient-stripped white flour. Way down the ingredient list, after water, was whole wheat flour. So, case closed: This was

The Many Different Identities of MSG

More than 40 different ingredients contain the chemical in MSG, *processed free glutamic acid*. Watch out for the following ingredients:

Monosodium glutamate; monopotassium glutamate; glutamate; anything else followed by "glutamate"; autolyzed yeast; calcium caseinate; sodium caseinate; gelatin; glutamic acid; yeast extract; anything "hydrolyzed"; "hydrolyzed protein" anything; calcium caseinate; sodium caseinate; yeast food; yeast nutrient; gelatin; textured protein; soy protein; soy protein concentrate; soy protein isolate; whey protein, whey protein concentrate; whey isolate; vetsin; ajinomoto.

not whole wheat bread, but white bread looking to disguise itself as whole wheat bread. (See The "Whole" Grain Truth below for how to solve the whole grain mystery and make sure the products you're putting in your cart are whole wheat.)

- **"All natural":** The FDA has issued several warning letters to firms making misleading "all natural" claims; however, the agency has never issued formal regulations about the term (except in the case of meat). As a result, some products containing high-fructose corn syrup, for example, claim to be "all natural." The term has no nutritional meaning whatsoever and is not regulated by the FDA in any foods except meat and poultry. When I see the phrase "all natural" on a box, bag, jar, or can, I simply dismiss it and move on to the ingredient list.

- **"No trans fat":** Many food products claim to have no trans fat. But thanks to an FDA labeling loophole, those claims are often untrue. Here's the dealio: The FDA allows food manufacturers to round to zero any ingredient that accounts for less than 0.5 grams per serving. So, a product claiming to have no trans fat can legally contain up to 0.5 grams per serving. While this might seem like a small amount, it's not; over time this small fraction adds up. Any amount of trans fat—even trace quantities—can increase your chances of developing heart disease. And it's super important to understand that when a food item contains trans fat, it's listed as "partially hydrogenated vegetable oil" in the ingredient list. Partially hydrogenated vegetable oil equals trans fat. Other phrases signifying trans fat are "hydrogenated oil," "vegetable shortening," "shortening," and "margarine."

The "Whole" Grain Truth

Most people think that "wheat flour" is the same thing as *whole grain* wheat flour. It's not. The confusion is exactly what the food industry wants. Food manufacturers are replacing the phrase "white flour" with the healthier sounding "wheat flour" because consumers have become aware of the negative consequences of eating white flour, a refined carb.

In reality, "wheat flour" is the exact same thing as "white flour." So "wheat flour" or "enriched wheat flour" is refined, processed wheat that's stripped of its nutritional value.

Another labeling trick, as I noted above, is the use of the phrase "made with whole grains!" on the front of packaging. Consumers see this and assume they're making a whole grain choice. What this term really means is that 5 percent of the product's ingredients are whole grains. Unfortunately, all this label trickery works. In a study done on the issue, 73 percent of moms mistakenly believed that "wheat flour" was the same as "whole-grain wheat flour." Below you will find all of the guidance you need to figure out when a product is truly a good source of whole grain.

A product is truly whole grain when it says:

- **100 percent whole grain** or **100 percent whole wheat**: This means the product contains zero refined white flour. This is the gold standard.

- **Whole grain**: probably contains little or no refined white flour. But check the ingredient list; if the first ingredient listed is "whole grain," then most likely this product is a winner. However, if it says "enriched wheat flour" or "stone ground flour" or any of the phrases below, it's a refined carb loser.

The following ingredients and phrases mean the product was made with refined grains, not whole grains.

• All-purpose flour	• Made with whole grain
• Bleached flour	• Stone ground flour
• Bread flour	• 12 grain (or multigrain)
• Cake flour	• Wheat flour
• Enriched wheat flour	• White flour
• Good source of whole grain	• Whole grain white flour

Because figuring out whether a product is a good source of whole grain is so confusing, the Whole Grains Council, a nonprofit consumer advocacy group, has created an official packaging symbol—the Whole

A Few of My Favorite Grains

Here are six whole grains or whole grain flours to try and what to do with them.

Amaranth: This grain is a yellow-gold seed that has a crunchy texture. It softens just a little when cooked. It's best mixed with other grains when you're making a pilaf or casserole. You can toast amaranth seeds and they'll expand just like popcorn.

Barley: This is a nutty flavored whole grain that is most commonly sold as pearled barley. Pearled barley is made from barley grains that have been split but still contain the pearl (center). Quaker Oats sells quick-cooking barley that can be made in 10 minutes. Barley is great in soups, salads, and simply on its own with some fresh herbs and vegetables such as mushrooms and zucchini.

Oats: This grain is probably the most popular grain in the world. There are several varieties of oats. Oatmeal is made from whole grain oats that have been stripped of their outer coating, steamed, rolled flat, and then thinly sliced. It is typically called old-fashioned oats or quick-cook oats. Steel-cut oats are not processed; they are nuttier and firmer than old-fashioned oats. Steel-cut oats produce creamier oatmeal but they take longer to cook, usually about 30 minutes. A quicker way to make steel-cut oats is to soak them overnight, at a ratio of ½ cup oats to 1½ cups water, with 1 tablespoon of an acid, such as vinegar, whey, kefir, or lemon juice. The next morning, simply add one more cup of water and cook for approximately 10 minutes. Quick-cook steel-cut oats are available at Trader Joe's, and they taste delicious.

Quinoa: Pronounced KEEN-wah, it has a very nutty flavor and pearly appearance. This grain is probably my favorite because it cooks in 10–15 minutes and can be used in a savory or sweet dish or substituted for oatmeal for breakfast. See my recipe for Asian Quinoa Salad on page 222.

Spelt: A great version of this grain is spelt flour, which can be used in place of wheat flour in recipes and can be tolerated by folks who have wheat allergies. It's my favorite nonwheat flour.

Wild rice: Believe it or not, this is technically not a rice but a tall aquatic grass. It can be used in soups, salads, casseroles, and stuffing.

Grain Stamp—to help you distinguish the real whole grain products from the chaff. The stamp started to appear on store shelves in 2005 and is becoming more widespread every day. However, and this is very important to keep in mind, many whole grain products are not yet using the stamp, so if a product doesn't have the stamp it might still be whole grain. You just have to default to the guidance laid out above.

There are two stamps in use. One, the 100 percent Stamp, assures you that a food contains a full serving or more of whole grain in each labeled serving and that *all* the grain is whole grain, while the basic Whole Grain Stamp appears on products containing at least half a serving of whole grain per serving.

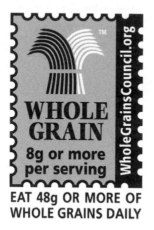

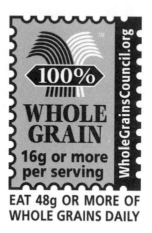

The Diet Food Aisle: Getting Fat on "Diet" Foods

In the past 4 decades, Americans got fat on "diet" foods. First, a tidal wave of "fat free," "no/low cholesterol," and "lite" products hit the supermarket shelves, then "carb free," "low carb," and "sugar free" labeling became all the rage. So what's wrong with these products? Read on.

FAT FREE, LITE, LOW CHOLESTEROL, NO CHOLESTEROL

Taking the fat out of foods doesn't magically make them nonfattening. In fact, many products contain copious amounts of sugar and salt to make up for the loss of flavor from removing or leaving out fat. Remember, fat adds flavor and texture to foods. In addition to loading up foods with added sugar and salt, manufacturers add other ingredients to enhance the taste. For instance, if you look at cream cheese, the regular version and its fat-free counterpart, you'll see that the fat-free cream cheese has twice as many ingredients. Emulsifiers are added to get the ingredients to stick together, and thickeners are used to mitigate the watery consistency. These fat stand-ins are not necessarily healthier than fat.

In addition to all of the unhealthy additives that go into these "diet" foods and their tricky labeling, companies take advantage of our fear of fat by charging more for these supposedly "healthier" foods.

As for the "low cholesterol" label, it's based on a dangerous myth that's been perpetuated for decades. That myth goes something like this: If you eat too much cholesterol, or saturated fat, your blood cholesterol will rise to dangerous levels. Excess cholesterol will then seep through your artery walls, causing thickenings or plaques that will eventually block blood flow in vital arteries, resulting in heart attacks and strokes. This myth has driven food manufacturers to extract cholesterol from cheese, eggs, and sausages. So for decades "low cholesterol" products like margarine and "light" foods have been considered healthy.

The truth, which is backed by a mountain of research, is there's no connection whatsoever between cholesterol in food and cholesterol in blood. Therefore, lowering cholesterol either through low-fat or low-cholesterol diets does not lower the risk of developing heart disease. And, as you've learned, the problem with margarine and other low-fat, low-cholesterol substitutes goes beyond the fact that they don't work to stop heart disease. In fact, as the consumption of real animal fats began to decrease and the consumption of supposedly healthy trans fats increased, the incidence of heart attacks began to rise.

All that said, there are a handful of food companies that are focused on providing real food products. For instance, if you read the ingredients on most brands of "low-fat" cheese you will learn quickly that they are indeed "real foods" with few, natural ingredients: skim milk, salt, cultures, and enzymes—all perfectly real and whole, but lower in saturated fats. The Strauss Family Creamery in California, for instance, offers lower-fat alternatives, such as Strauss's skim milk, that don't contain additives or added sugar to make up for the fat that's left out. So, sometimes a product that markets the fact that it's a lower-fat alternative is genuine. It's just a matter of reading the ingredients, and knowing what you're eating, not just what you aren't.

CAR FREE, LOW-CARB, SUGAR FREE

As is the case with fat-free diet foods, the problem with carb free/ low-carb/sugar free foods is what is added to the foods to make up for what's been taken out. In this case, the add-ins are typically sugar alcohols. Erythritol, isomalt, lactiol, mannitol, malitol, sorbitol, and xylitol are all sugar alcohols. And humans lack the enzymes to break them down. As a result, if you eat too much food containing them, you might suffer gastrointestinal distress, like bloating, gas, or abdominal pain. However, I feel it is important to note that there are documented human studies on erythritol and xylitol that show these sweeteners do not cause any GI distress when eaten in moderation. I use ZSweet, a combination of stevia and erythritol, in some of the recipes in this book.

Perhaps the most insidious outcome of eating all of these "diet" foods is that we end up overeating them, for a couple of reasons. For one thing, psychologically we think of them as "guilt-free" and give ourselves permission to eat more. And for another, because of all the factory additives, they're just not as satisfying as real food. At the end of the day, a better route is to go on a diet food-free diet and simply eat smaller portions of healthy real food.

Nutrition Facts: Label Reading 101

In Chapter 8, I told you that whenever I purchase a food item from the supermarket, I always read the ingredients label first. If the list passes muster, the next step is to read the nutrition label to make sure it too checks out.

Starting below, I'm going to go through the different components of the label and give you some general guidelines as to what you should be on the lookout for.

Nutrition Facts

Serving Size 1/2 cup (about 82g)
Servings Per Container 8

Amount Per Serving

Calories 200   Calories from Fat 130

		% Daily Value*
Total Fat 14g		**22%**
Saturated Fat 9g		**45%**
Trans Fat 0g		
Cholesterol 55mg		**18%**
Sodium 40mg		**2%**
Total Carbohydrate 17g		**6%**
Dietary Fiber 1g		**4%**
Sugars 14g		
Protein 3g		

Vitamin A 10%   •   Vitamin C 0%

Calcium 10%   •   Iron 6%

*Percent Daily Values are based on a 2,000 calorie diet. Your daily values may be higher or lower depending on your calorie needs:

		Calories: 2,000	2,500
Total Fat	Less than	65g	80g
Saturated Fat	Less than	20g	25g
Cholesterol	Less than	300mg	300 mg
Sodium	Less than	2,400mg	2,400mg
Total Carbohydrate		300g	375g
Dietary Fiber		25g	30g

- **Serving size:** This tells you what amount of the food or drink the nutritional information is based on. Some nutrition panels will also tell you how many servings are in the package or container. Look carefully at the serving size. There may be 2, 3, or more servings in the package, which obviously doubles or triples the number of calories and the amounts of the ingredients in the food if you eat the whole thing.

- **Calories:** As a general rule, you should stick to 300 to 500 calories in one meal if you intend to lose weight. That being said, in my opinion the number of calories in a serving of food is not as critical as the amount of protein, carbs, fats, and real-food ingredients. In this book I teach you to eat to stabilize blood sugar levels, so the focus should not be so much on calories as on how you are balancing your carbs with your protein and fats. If the food has 70 grams of carbs but just 4 grams of protein, that food will definitely spike blood sugar, so I recommend you avoid it.

- **Total fat:** Total fat tells you how much fat is in a serving. Some labels, like the one shown, do break out saturated and trans fat and give the amounts of each. But just as many do not. The reason is the food industry does not want to call attention to the fact that their products contain trans fat. Therefore, many labels will simply list the total amount of fat and then break out and list the total amount of saturated fat leaving it up to you to do your detective work on the ingredients list to figure out what other kinds of fat the product contains. Avoid foods with more than 15 grams of fat per serving if you would like to lose weight (unless you are sure it is a "good" fat).

- **Cholesterol:** Too much cholesterol means the food is high in fat. Remember, you want to keep your fat intake to a ballpark of 40 grams a day (10 grams per meal) for weight loss.

- **Sodium:** You really need to be diligent in reducing your sodium intake. By the USDA's reckoning, a food is low in sodium if it contains no more than 140 milligrams per serving. As a rule, the amount of sodium should be less than double the number of calories per serving.

- **Total carbohydrates:** This category includes everything from whole grains to sugar and other refined carbs. Typically, a nutrition panel will break down the carbohydrate total, detailing how much fiber and sugar is included in the total number.

- **Sugar, Sugar, SUGAR!** This number is super important. In fact, this is one of the major bits of information that I hope will make an imprint on your brain and never go away. When it comes to the sugar count on a nutrition label, the most important information you need to know is that

     4 grams of nutrition label sugar = 1 actual teaspoon of sugar

     I don't want you to go crazy counting grams of sugar, but if your goal is to lose weight, aim for no more than 5 teaspoons, or

Beware of Added Sugar!

The following table, which was put together by the American Heart Association, shows how many teaspoons of added sugar a person should eat, according to the USDA's current nutrition recommendations.

DAILY CALORIES	TEASPOONS OF ADDED SUGAR
1200	4
1400	4
1600	3
1800	5
2000	8
2200	9
2400	12
2600	14
2800	15
3000	18*

*The recommended number of teaspoons of added sugar decreases for 1600 calories because that amount represents a calorie recommendation for young children ages 4 to 8 years of age. To accommodate all of the food groups to meet nutrient requirements for this age group, fewer calories are available for a discretionary calorie allowance, according to the AHA.

According to the American Heart Association, the average American consumes more than 22 teaspoons of sugar a day—way more than the numbers on this chart. We're talking about sugars that are added to foods during manufacturing or processing, not naturally occurring sugars in fruits and vegetables. So if you're on a 2,000 calorie a day diet, the AHA says it's okay for you to eat 8 teaspoons of added sugar a day. If you're the average American, you're eating 14 teaspoons more than that. That's a lot of sugar!

20 grams, of added sugars per day. Remember that natural sugars are okay to consume in a healthy PC (protein-carb) or FC (fat-carb) combo. The villain is too many added sugars, which can be found in even seemingly healthy foods like yogurts.

- **Protein:** On this real-food diet, between 20 percent and 25 percent of your total calories should come from protein. That comes out to about 20–22 grams of protein per meal. Remember, it is important to also look at how many grams of carbs and fat your food has. Generally you want your meal to be approximately one part protein to two parts carbohydrates and under 15 grams of good fats.

Why Organic Isn't Necessarily Healthy

The popularity of organic foods has grown astronomically in the past couple of decades. In the U.S., sales of organic food have grown from $1 billion in 1990 to $24.8 billion in 2009, according to the Organic Trade Association. Consumer demand for organic food has attracted large corporations to the organic marketplace. Major corporations are now responsible for at least 25 percent of all organic manufacturing and marketing (40 percent if you count only processed organic foods). As a result, much of the nation's organic food is now, unfortunately, a product of factory food manufacturing.

At the core of the organic farming philosophy is the desire to return the nutrients that are lost in the growing process back to the soil. This philosophy also calls for raising animals humanely in accordance with nature. It's meant to result in the production of the most nutritious food possible. However, the government regulations that mandate what foods can or can't be labeled "organic" aren't that stringent, and allow some questionable practices.

For instance, under the regulations, animals whose meat is certified "organic" must be given access to the outdoors, but for how long and under what conditions is not spelled out. The common "cage free" and "free range" labels may lead consumers to imagine a picturesque pastoral setting, but that's not the norm. Rather, it often means that a relatively small patio with a cement floor, and no grass or dirt flooring, has been added on to the structure where the animals are kept.

Furthermore, while it's true that animals that produce organic foods can't be given antibiotics or hormones, there's no requirement that they be fed what they're meant to eat in nature. For example, cattle that produce certified organic beef may be fed organic grains instead of their natural diet of grass. This affects the animal's health and is detrimental to the nutritional quality of the meat.

When it comes to processed foods, consumers automatically assume they are healthy just because they bear the "certified organic" label. This thinking is misguided. Think about it: A bag of organic potato chips, having come from organic potatoes, might be free of pesticide, but at the end of the day, they're still fried in unhealthy processed oil and full of added salt. And the organic version of Pop Tarts, "toaster pastries," is just as loaded with processed fat and refined carbs. As Marion Nestle says, "Organic junk food is still junk food."

USDA Certified Organic

The primary organic certification you will see is "USDA Organic." The United States Department of Agriculture (USDA) sets forth requirements that must be met before a farmer or food producer can use its certified organic emblem. Its soil is tested and must have been free of chemical exposure for at least 3 years. The food it produces must be free of any chemical or genetically engineered ingredients and must not have been raised or produced with any drugs or hormones. It also can't be irradiated.

Although in some cases the label of a certified organic product specifies that it's 100 percent organic, the USDA requires that only 95 percent of a certified organic product's ingredients actually be organic. The remaining 5 percent do not have to be organic. The USDA's list of allowed substances for the remaining 5 percent includes more than 200 nonorganic and synthetic items. Foods with the label "made with organic ingredients" must contain between 70 percent and 94 percent organic ingredients. Products with less than 70 percent organic ingredients may list organic ingredients only on the information panel of the packaging. Neither may bear the USDA Organic seal.

Even if a producer is certified organic, the use of the USDA Organic label is voluntary. Not everyone who produces organic foods chooses to go through the rigorous and expensive process of becoming certified organic. This is especially true for smaller farming operations. For example, when shopping at your local farmers' market, don't hesitate to ask vendors how their food is grown. They often use organic practices but are not USDA certified organic. I buy much of my food from growers who are in this category.

Certified Naturally Grown

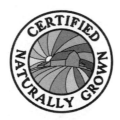

Some of the highest quality foods may come from farmers who haven't gone through the USDA's certification process. Case in point: the "Certified Naturally Grown" (CNG) label. The CNG label is a nonprofit farm assurance certification program created for small-scale organic farmers who are striving to strengthen the organic movement by preserving high organic standards and removing financial barriers that tend to exclude smaller farms that sell locally and directly to their customers.

CNG farmers follow the USDA standards of the National Organic Program, but the recordkeeping and inspection process is tailored to accommodate the needs of small-scale mixed-agriculture farmers who are not normally permitted to use the word "organic." Farmers commit to act as inspectors. Inspection forms are posted on the Internet for public access, and all farms are subject to random pesticide residue testing. All in all, the CNG procedure requires less paperwork yet, many argue, results in more transparency and fosters better farming practices than organic certification does. The reasoning is that CNG depends on farmer-inspectors who are uniquely qualified to observe and note whether their colleagues are adhering to the standards. Plus, the interaction between the farmer-inspectors and the farmers fosters a sharing of information that in the end results in the creation of a sense of community. On the other hand, USDA Organic is a bureaucratic program that inspects mountains of paperwork rather than the actual farm.

Despite the flaws in the USDA Organic label, having the option available is certainly better than not having the option. But, bottom line: you shouldn't trust the USDA Organic label blindly. Instead, you must take responsibility for your health and commit yourself to finding reputable sources of high quality food. What's more, the American diet is so abysmal that, as my favorite real-food activist Mark Bittman puts it, "The organic question is a secondary one. It's not unimportant, but it's not the primary issue in the way Americans eat."

The Meat and Poultry Department: Label Says What?!

Meat is the only product sold in the U.S. that comes with a government seal of approval. It was after Upton Sinclair's 1905 novel *The Jungle*, about the unsanitary practices of the meat industry, that the 1906 Federal Meat Inspection Act was passed into law. For nearly a century, that was the only label that mattered. But now, a slew of new labels on meat make more specific promises. Today's labels tackle consumer concerns about the living conditions and diets of the animals. Some of the claims are backed by USDA authority and have concrete definitions; some are monitored by animal rights or environmental groups; some are created by businesses themselves, which employ private auditors to guarantee compliance with their criteria. A few of these labels are more than just marketing, as the USDA has some strict rules about who can use certain labels. Below is a list that defines what most of the more common labels you read on meat really mean.

I recommend steering clear of meat that comes from a CAFO and buying meat that is raised as humanely and naturally as possible. The healthiest meat is from animals that eat a natural diet and haven't been raised in unsanitary, overcrowded living conditions—for instance, cows that are pasture raised or grass fed; chickens and pigs that are free-range and allowed to peck and forage for their food. This meat is free of antibiotics and growth hormones and high in omega-3 fats. That said, the Real-Food Movement is still in its early days, so this meat isn't currently available to everyone, everywhere, at an affordable price. Someday it will be, but the reality is that we're just not there yet. So my advice to you is to do your best to buy the healthiest meat you can. If it's at all possible for you to buy free range, grass fed, pasture raised meat, do it. If you can't, buy as clean as you can. The explanations of the meat labels below will help you to do that.

Organic: In order to give its official certified organic label, the USDA must verify that the animal was given pesticide- and chemical fertilizer-free food and never given hormones or antibiotics—ever. Meat from animals treated with antibiotics for illness cannot be sold as organic, even if the animals recover to full health. Organic meat has to be processed (slaughtered and butchered) in a certified organic facility.

Natural: "Natural" is perhaps the most misleading label on meat. The USDA defines "natural" and "all natural" food products as those that have been minimally processed and contain no preservatives or artificial ingredients. Since this is true of all fresh meat, this label is relatively meaningless.

No hormones (beef): First of all, there is no such thing as a "hormone-free" animal. All animals have hormones naturally. But because cattle are often given synthetic hormones to promote growth, there is a

USDA label for beef grown without these hormones. Keep in mind that it's against federal regulations to treat pork and poultry with hormones, so never pay more for that label on a chicken.

No antibiotics (red meat and poultry) *(not always reliable)*: In the U.S., animals raised in crowded conditions are often treated with antibiotics to prevent illness and to help promote rapid growth. For meat and poultry, the USDA has defined "no antibiotics administered" to mean that the animal was raised without low-level or therapeutic doses of antibiotics. Unless there is an organization identified as a third-party certifier, there is no organization backing the claim other than the producer. This claim is approved by the USDA based on documentation provided by the producer.

Grass fed *(not always reliable)*: USDA regulated. It means, very narrowly, that animals eat grass. According to the USDA definition, "grass fed" animals can also be fed grain and can be raised on grass in confinement, as long as they have access to pasture. As documented in *The Omnivore's Dilemma*, by Michael Pollan, and elsewhere, "access" can be—and often is—nothing more than a facility with a door to a small outdoor area. Livestock are transferred to this facility after they have been conditioned to remain indoors in a facility with no such exit. The program is voluntary, however, without third-party verification. Labels that read "100 percent grass fed" or "grass-finished" and verified by a third party, such as the American Grassfed Association, will guarantee the beef has fed only grass and hay. The "USDA Process Verified Grass Fed" label indicates that cattle and other ruminant animals were fed only grass, hay, and other forages and had continuous

Are Processed Meats Bad for Me?

Many cured and processed meats contain nitrates, a preservative that can be carcinogenic. A 2010 study in the journal *Cancer*, for instance, showed nitrates in cold cuts increased risk for bladder cancer. In addition, high sodium levels in processed meats contribute to hypertension and weight loss-stalling water retention. They also often contain fillers and artificial colors.

access to the outdoors during the growing season. A "grass fed" label that does not include the words "USDA Process Verified" means the producer's claim was evaluated by the USDA but not verified by the agency through on-site inspection.

Free range: "Free range" suggests that a meat or poultry product (including eggs) came from an animal that was able to roam outdoors. However, the USDA regulates the term "free range" only for poultry, not for beef or eggs, and birds are required only to have access to the outdoors, which could be a concrete feedlot. The USDA considers 5 minutes of outdoor time each day to be sufficient. This claim is not verified by an independent third party.

Cage free *(not reliable)*: Commonly seen on egg cartons, "cage free" indicates that eggs come from chickens or other poultry that were not

Meat and Poultry in
U.S. Antibiotic Resistant

Most food animals are raised in crowded CAFOs (confined animal feeding operations) and fed grain grown with chemical fertilizers and pesticides. To promote faster growth and compensate for unhealthy conditions, CAFOs add antibiotics to animal feed—accounting for about 70 percent of all antibiotics and related drugs used in the U.S. This overuse of antibiotics leads to the development of antibiotic-resistant diseases that are more difficult and expensive to treat for both the animals receiving the antibiotics and the humans eating them. Meat and poultry produced in the United States is widely contaminated with "multi-drug-resistant" bacteria, according to a study published in April 2011. The report, published in the April 15 edition of *Clinical Infectious Diseases*, found that nearly half of the samples of poultry and meat in the study were contaminated with bacteria. Slightly more than half of the contaminated samples, one out of four in all, were resistant to various antibiotics, according to the study. The samples were collected from 26 grocery stores in Chicago; Fort Lauderdale, Florida; Los Angeles; Washington, D.C.; and Flagstaff, Arizona.

confined in cages, but the label is not highly regulated by the USDA. "Cage free" does not necessarily mean that the birds were raised with adequate space or that they had access to the outdoors.

Certified humane raised and handled *(reliable)*: Humane Farm Animal Care, an independent nonprofit organization, certifies eggs, dairy, meat, and poultry. Its Animal Care Standards require that animals be allowed to engage in their natural behaviors, have sufficient space, shelter, and gentle handling to limit stress, and have ample fresh water and a healthy diet without added antibiotics or hormones. This type of label wards against practices like overcrowding, castrating, early weaning, and denying animals access to pasture. Inspections are carried out annually.

Demeter Certified Biodynamic® *(reliable)*: The concept of Biodynamic® farming, developed in the 1920s, views the farm holistically as a living organism and emphasizes contributing to natural resources instead of depleting them. Biodynamic® products must be produced without synthetic pesticides or fertilizers or genetic engineering and meet all other requirements of a certified organic label. When meat is labeled Biodynamic®, there were no animal by-products used in the livestock feed.

Pasture raised: This usually means that the animal spent most of its life feeding in an open pasture rather than in a feedlot. However, there are not official standards for this label yet.

Local: Producers who take part in this affidavit program state in writing that the animals were raised within 20 miles of where they are being sold. This label is not certified (or confirmed) by a third party, such as the USDA or a labeling certifier.

Grass finished: This can mean anything from cattle fed exclusively grass to cattle raised on corn and then fed grass during the last few weeks before slaughter.

100 percent vegetarian diet: Not certified by an independent organization. Producers will say this to indicate that the livestock or poultry was not fed any animal by-products, but only hay, grass, or grains; however, there is no guarantee that it is actually true. This label does not signify that the animal was raised on a pasture.

Nutrition Labels on Meat

The Agriculture Department will require many meat labels to include the number of calories and other nutritional information starting in 2012 so that consumers can make healthier decisions about what they eat. The requirement will apply to 40 of the most popular cuts of meat and poultry products. Ground meat and poultry will have the facts on their labels. Raw cuts will offer the information on labels or to consumers at the point of purchase.

Labels will list grams of total fat and saturated fat, and fat percentages for products already offering lean percentages. The main cuts affected are boneless chicken breasts, brisket, and tenderloin steak. The rule also affects hamburger and ground turkey. So now we'll have a more accurate way to ensure that we're buying lean meat. And when it comes to weight loss, the leaner the meat the better.

The Seafood Counter

As I told you in Chapter 4, seafood is an amazing source of good omega-3 fats. Fish with darker flesh, such as salmon, mackerel, herring, trout, and others are among the best seafood sources of omega-3 fats. The benefits of fish and seafood are so great that the government's recently released 2010 *Dietary Guidelines for Americans* recommend that Americans increase their seafood intake to at least 8 ounces a week, or about 2 servings. The guidelines, from the U.S. Department of Agriculture and the Department of Health and Human Services, say adults now consume only about $3^1/_2$ ounces a week.

When it comes to choosing fish at the fish counter, I recommend choosing wild raised rather than farmed. Fish farming presents many of the same problems that factory livestock farming does: pollution, unsanitary and inhumane living conditions for the fish, an inferior final food product, and a threat to the natural balance of our planet's ecosystem. A typical fish farm may cram up to 90,000 fish in a single pen that's 100 feet long by 100 feet wide. Many of the fish species are also fed an unnatural diet. They often eat pellets made of wheat, soy, antibiotics, pesticides, and hormones. So instead of getting a healthy dose of omega-3s when eating seafood raised in this way, you get an unneeded dose of omega-6s, which you don't need and which contributes to an uneven balance of omegas.

Farm raised fish contain even more of the pollutants that are a problem with all seafood: mercury and PCBs. Farmed fish also contain lower levels of vitamins A and D than their wild counterparts, because of their diets. Unfortunately, a large majority of the fish that's available in restaurants and supermarkets is farm raised and should ideally be avoided unless you can verify that it's fresh caught. (Farm raised clams and oysters are not raised using the same practices as fish. I do order them from restaurants and I eat them with zest!) Even "organic" farm raised fish isn't much better. Organic fish farmers follow many of the same flawed practices as conventional fish farmers, including the use of overcrowded pens and unnatural feed.

HOW TO BUY SAFE SEAFOOD

I've read, researched, and interviewed experts on this matter, and I will tell you, it's an extremely complicated topic, and it's terribly difficult to come up with a consensus. Nonetheless, here are the rules that I myself follow, and that I am comfortable passing along to you.

- Only eat wild caught fish. (Again, you can use more leeway with oysters and clams.)

- One merchant I trust to buy frozen salmon from is Vital Choice Wild Seafood & Organics. The seafood from Vital Choice is from remote Alaskan waters and is randomly tested to verify minimal levels of contamination.

- I consider Target, Wegmans, and Whole Foods to be reliable stores from which to buy seafood as they have adopted seafood sustainability practices far more effectively than many other major retailers. (Read "On Eating Sustainable Fish," an article written by real-food advocate Mark Bittman, published April 7, 2010, in the *New York Times*. It's fantastic and further explains this issue.) I always consult the online source Monterey Bay Aquarium before I go shopping for seafood to see what kind of seafood it recommends at the moment from both a health and an environmental standpoint. (Overfishing is a huge environmental concern, and for some this carries weight in their decision-making.) Just log on to its Web site at www.montereybayaquarium.org and click on the Seafood Watch link in the lower right-hand corner. Then click on Seafood Recommendation in the left-hand navigation. From there, scroll down and you will see the Our Seafood Ratings box.

Going this route ensures you get a selection of seafood that's both good for you and good for the planet. Or you can download the site's Seafood Watch Guide, which lists dozens of seafood species, and check to see what the ratings are for the different fish listed. Below are the seafood ratings.

- **Best Choices:** Seafood in this category is abundant, well managed, and caught or farmed in environmentally friendly ways.
- **Good Alternatives:** These items are an option, but there are concerns about how they're caught or farmed or about the quality of their habitat.
- **Avoid:** Take a pass on these items for now. They are caught or farmed in ways that harm other marine life or the environment.
- **The Super Green List:** A list of wild and farmed seafood that's healthy for people and the oceans.

Clicking on The Super Green List will bring you to a list of seafood that meets the following criteria:

- Low levels of contaminants (less than 216 parts per billion [ppb] mercury and less than 11 ppb PCBs)
- The daily minimum of omega-3s (at least 250 milligrams per day [mg/d])*
- Classified as a Seafood Watch Best Choice (in green)

It's super easy to use the site; trust me, after you use it once you'll totally get the hang of it. Also, the Seafood Watch Guide is now available as a free app for your iPod or iPhone. Just search for "seafood watch" in the App Store.

*Dietary requirements for an average woman of childbearing age (18–45, 154 pounds) eating 8 ounces of fish per week. The list also applies to men and children; children should eat age-appropriate portions to maximize their health benefits while minimizing risk. The recommendation of 250 mg of omega-3s refers to the combined level of two omega-3s of primary importance to human health: eicosapentanoic acid (EPA) and docosahexaenoic acid (DHA).

When I can remember that a certain fish is troubled—most cod, for example, and bluefin tuna, and most species of shark and skate—either from a health or an environmental standpoint, I don't buy it.

Produce Department

Food that comes from plants is the foundation of a real-food diet. A great way to make sure you're getting all the nutrients produce has to offer is to make a concerted effort to eat a variety of different colors. Each group, as you'll see, contains nutrients that not only help you lose weight but also keep you healthy.

GREEN

Arugula, bok choy, broccoli, broccolini, broccoli rabe, broccoli sprouts, Brussels sprouts, cabbage, collard greens, kale, mustard greens, rutabaga, Swiss chard, turnip greens, turnips, watercress

This group of vegetables is called cruciferous because their flowers often bloom in the shape of a cross. They contain a variety of healthful compounds, one of which has been shown to increase detoxification of estrogen in the liver by as much as 50 percent. This is a big deal during weight loss, when the liver is inundated with estrogen-like chemicals from your fat stores.

Note: Large amounts of raw cruciferous vegetables on a daily basis can impair thyroid function, so it's best to have most of them cooked.

PURPLE AND RED

Beets, blackberries, black currants, blueberries, cherries, cranberries, eggplant, plums, pomegranates, purple cabbage, raspberries, red apples, strawberries

This color group is most noted for its water-soluble antioxidants, called anthocyanins, which help reduce the risk of cancer, heart disease, diabetes, allergies, DNA damage, inflammation, and premature aging. They also support the production of adiponectin, a hormone that suppresses appetite, helps burn body fat, and reduces the risk of diabetes.

In my opinion, blueberries are the superstar of this group because they are one of the highest in antioxidants of any fruit or vegetable. Blueberries contain phytochemical anthocyanidins and are rich in pectin, a fiber that binds to toxins. Another bonus: Blueberries have a compound, similar to the one found in cranberries, that helps prevent urinary tract infections.

Raspberries also deserve a shout-out when it comes to weight loss. According to a Japanese study, raspberries have unique weight loss effects. Researchers isolated a compound in raspberries that helped laboratory animals reduce abdominal fat, triglycerides, total body fat, and overall weight, and improved their ability to burn fat.

ORANGE, YELLOW, AND GREEN

Vegetables: bell peppers, carrots, green beans, leafy greens, lettuce, green peas, peppers, pumpkin, spinach, squash, sweet potatoes, tomatoes, zucchini

Fruits: apricots, cantaloupes, clementines, grapefruits, guava, honeydew, kiwi, lemons, nectarines, oranges, passion fruit, peaches, pears, persimmons, tangerines, watermelon

This group is best known for its fat-soluble phytonutrients called carotenoids. They are also very high in vitamin C. The fruits and vegetables in this group range from yellow to green because the chlorophyll that gives plants their characteristic green color can overshadow orange pigment in certain foods.

These fruits and vegetables help increase insulin sensitivity, prevent stress-related weight gain in the abdomen, and protect our cells from toxin damage during weight loss.

WHITE

Chives, endives, garlic, leeks, onions, scallions, shallots

The members of this group are known as alliums because they contain a powerful phytonutrient called allicin. Allicin has been shown to help lower blood pressure, prevent cancer, improve sensitivity of cells to insulin and leptin (the satiety hormone), and destroy yeast in the intestines. Allicin also helps with detoxification by increasing the production of glutathione (an antioxidant naturally produced by our bodies), which helps eliminate toxins and carcinogenic substances from the body.

The Dairy Aisle—Milk: Got Controversy?

Milk is perhaps one of the most controversial foods in the American diet. To make sure you're getting the healthiest option in your basket, I'm going to answer four of the most important questions about milk.

Do humans need to drink milk for strong bones?

For decades our government and the powerful dairy industry have told us milk is good for us. Here's what the USDA says about milk: "[Dairy products] provide high-quality protein and are good sources of vitamins A, D, and B-12, and also riboflavin, phosphorus, magnesium, potassium, zinc and calcium." This is true. Today milk provides more than 70 percent of the calcium in the American diet, and is fortified with vitamin D to prevent rickets. The USDA tells us to eat 3 servings of dairy foods a day. Sounds simple enough.

But as with everything else we eat these days, it's a heck of a lot more complicated than it seems. Dairy milk itself is a complex substance. Cows produce it for their young, and it's the perfect food—for calves. But why is milk is supposed to be so good for you?

The major marketing push has always revolved around milk as a good source of calcium. Cow's milk is indeed high in calcium; however, whether a diet high in dairy calcium protects you against osteoporosis or any other disease is highly contestable. Calcium is the major chemical element that makes up our bones, and we need to take in calcium to replace the amount that is lost through normal turnover in our bone cells. As Marion Nestle, one of the most trusted nutritionists in the U.S., points out, though, while some of the components in cow's milk help us to hang on to calcium in our bodies, other components cause us to let go of calcium. Plus, successful calcium turnover is not just dependent on us getting enough calcium, it also depends on how much you get of other key nutrients, how active you are, whether you smoke, and whether you drink a lot of alcohol.

So, in reality, getting enough calcium is just one piece of the big puzzle—and milk isn't the only or even necessarily the best source of calcium. In fact, in areas of the world where milk isn't a staple, people have fewer bone fractures and the incidence of osteoporosis is much lower. These folks get half the calcium intake that we do and their calcium balance is fine. Plus, as Marion Nestle notes, cows stop drinking the stuff after calfhood, but they're able to grow bones strong enough to support their 800-plus pounds of body weight. Cows eat grass (or at least they're supposed to), and grass contains calcium (as does every other food from plants, including fruits, veggies, grains, beans, and nuts) as well as the other nutrients we need to help us absorb the calcium, like magnesium.

So, the answer to the question is "no." Although our government, with the encouragement of a very powerful dairy industry lobbying effort, pushes us to drink our milk, milk is not a nutritional requirement. It's just one food choice in a world full of food choices. It's not a super-food and it's not the end-all, be-all of maintaining bone strength. In fact, it has some major downsides to it, such as the fact that it's extremely high in fat and cholesterol, both of which are bad in large amounts, and it has a sugar in it, lactose, which many people over the age of 5 have trouble digesting. In addition, because of the current dairy farming methods, which are focused on getting more milk from fewer cows in the shortest amount of time, large amounts of hormones and antibiotics are given to milk-producing cows. Read on to gain an understanding of the effects of those substances.

Are the hormones and antibiotics in milk bad for us?

In 1970, each cow in the U.S. produced 9,700 pounds of milk per year; now, thanks to genetically engineered hormones, each produces nearly 20,000. One such hormone that's commonly given to dairy cows in this country is called rbST. Most likely, neither rbST nor the natural growth hormone it's patterned after, bST, is harmful to humans. Structurally, they're different from our own human growth hormones, so they don't activate in our bodies. Also, these hormones are proteins, so our stomach acids deactivate them like they do other proteins, and enzymes in our intestines break them down into amino acids. So the hormones themselves aren't dangerous. However, they do raise a host of safety issues due to the effect they have on the cows.

First, injecting cows regularly with rbST results in their being more at risk for infections, both at injection sites on their skin and because the more milk their udders produce, the more prone they are to udder infections. So the cows are regularly given antibiotics that can get into the milk. Once we drink the milk, those antibiotics can kill our bodies' friendly bacteria, setting us up for health issues, or they can cause bacteria that can harm us by making us become resistant to antibiotics. Dairies are supposed to keep antibiotics out of our milk supply, but the system in place to protect against this issue is hardly foolproof.

Omega-3 Source:
Organic Milk from Grass Fed Cows

Organic milk from grass fed cows contains higher levels of omega-3 fatty acids. Grass fed, pasture-roaming cows' milk contains up to 50 percent more omega-3 fats compared to factory farm cows, according to Dr. Jonny Bowden's *150 Healthiest Foods on Earth*. This is due to a natural diet rich in grass, insects, and soil.

The bigger concern behind the use of rbST is that giving cows this growth hormone increases the amount of so-called "insulin-like growth factor" (IGF-1) in their milk. A cow's IGF-1 is identical to the human form of IGF-1, so if you drink milk from cows treated with rbST, your own levels of IGF-1 could spike. IGF-1 is a protein and should be mostly obliterated by our stomach acid and intestinal enzymes, but there's always the chance that it will get absorbed intact. Health studies have linked high blood levels of IGF-1 to increased risks of prostate cancer in men and breast cancer in women.

The use of rbST is the reason that I do recommend the purchase of organic milk if you drink milk. In order to earn that certified organic label, the milk must come from cows that were given organic feed and can't be given antibiotics, except to treat disease, or hormones.

Are lower-fat milk options, like skim milk, bad for us?

Many real-foodies opt to drink whole milk instead of skim, low-fat, or reduced-fat milk. The reason behind their decision is twofold. One reason is that they are concerned that when the fat is removed, so is a portion of its nutritional quality. For example, when the fat is removed from milk so is most of the vitamin A, a fat-soluble vitamin. Another reason is that it's standard practice, as I told you in Chapter 2, for dairy producers to improve upon the rather watery consistency of skim milk and low-fat milk by adding dried milk powder to it. Dried milk is produced by forcing skim milk through tiny holes at high temperatures and pressures. This process causes the milk's cholesterol to become oxidized, and oxidized cholesterol has been linked to heart disease.

However, some nutrition experts, like Ed Blonz, a Ph.D. in nutrition science, counter that the amounts of oxidized cholesterol are so minimal that they do not pose a health risk, and that the loss of vitamin A is not a big deal in the total scheme of things because there are many other sources of vitamin A in our diets. For her part, nutritionist Marion Nestle asserts, "If you drink milk at all, the lower its fat content the better its nutritional value. Nonfat milk retains most of the nutrients in whole milk but hardly any of the calories or fat."

Armed with the different sides of the argument, it's up to you to decide where you stand. Personally, I don't drink milk because I am lactose intolerant, but I'm okay with my clients drinking either kind. I don't think you should shy away from whole milk, but if you are looking to drop pounds, switch to skim milk. Or, if you choose to drink only whole milk, just drink less of it, because there's one thing that is not up for discussion: Whole milk is high in fat and calories. And remember, if you're following the real-food diet, you'll need to make sure that any beverages you drink (whether it's skim milk, raw whole milk, or anything else) fit into the meal guidelines for the diet.

Does raw milk belong on the real food menu?

Before I let you in on my position on raw milk, I first want to give you a bit of background on the raw milk movement. Raw milk is milk that hasn't gone through pasteurization, a process of heating designed to destroy microorganisms that can cause spoilage and disease. In addition, raw milk is not homogenized. Homogenization breaks up fat globules into such a small size that they remain suspended. Raw milk, as it comes from the cow, is an emulsion, a mixture of milk fat globules, various solids, and water. Over time, the fat globules separate and rise to the surface as a layer of cream, leaving what is essentially skim milk below. In the years before homogenization, folks had to shake the milk to keep the cream mixed in.

Twenty years ago, the FDA banned interstate sales of unpasteurized milk. In 2007, the agency warned consumers that they were risking their health drinking raw milk. Many government officials and the majority of public health organizations hold to the need for pasteurization. Before pasteurization, many dairies, especially in cities, fed their cattle low-quality food, and their milk was rife with dangerous bacteria. Pasteurizing it was the only way to make it safe to drink. In 1938, milk caused 25 percent of all outbreaks of food- and water-related sickness. With the advent of pasteurization, that number fell to 1 percent by 1993, according to the Center for Science in the Public Interest. But individual states determine how raw milk is bought and sold within their borders. Twenty-eight states allow the sale of raw milk.

Advocates of raw milk in the U.S. make two basic arguments for it. They say that pasteurization destroys or damages some of the milk's nutrients, and that while pasteurization may kill dangerous bacteria, it also kills off beneficial, good bacteria, as well as proteins and enzymes. Advocates attribute stronger immune systems and better digestive systems to raw milk.

Here's what two of my go-to real-food gurus have to say, and to make matters interesting, they don't exactly agree.

Nina Planck, founder of London Farmers' Markets and author of Real Food: What to Eat and Why, *drank raw milk while she was pregnant and nursing. She is one of the country's leading champions for the cause of raw milk. Here's what she has to say: "So why do we drink raw milk even though there is a small chance we'll get sick? Well, I find first after doing all my research that I trust the traditional food chain more than I trust the industrial food chain. There are a number of risks from eating industrial food and I try to minimize and avoid those risks too. We drink raw milk simply because it's got more good food in it." Among the good food she's referring to are B vitamins; omega-3 fats; and enzymes including lipase, which helps you digest fats; phosphatase, which helps you absorb calcium; and lactase, which helps you digest lactose. All of these are damaged by pasteurization.*

Marion Nestle, on the other hand, states: "My position on raw milk has long been that people have a right to drink it but it had better be produced safely. But food safety experts tell me that raw milk can never be tested frequently enough to be confident it is safe. Raw milk carries a greater risk of bacterial contamination than pasteurized milk and . . . putting a child at risk of hemolytic uremic syndrome from toxic E. coli just doesn't make sense to me. . . . I'm dubious about the claims made for the health benefits of raw milk. No question, it tastes better and that may be reason enough to want it. But until I can be sure that the producer is scrupulous about safety, my personal choice favors pasteurization."

Although I am not opposed to raw milk on principle, I agree with Marion Nestle that it's important to know that the milk producer was scrupulous about safety. If I could see for myself that a raw milk producer had a well-designed and well-monitored safety system in place and was testing regularly for harmful bacteria, I would worry less about drinking it. In the meantime, I personally view pasteurization as a small price to pay for not having to worry about whether milk is safe to drink. But again, now that you know the facts, you should make the choice you feel most comfortable with.

Vat Pasteurization: A Happy Medium?

Unlike standard pasteurization, which is designed to handle huge volumes of milk at high temperatures, vat pasteurization heats the milk at lower temperatures but for a longer duration. As part of the process, the milk is held at 145°F for 30 minutes and then cooled as quickly as possible.

Proponents of this method say the milk is of a higher quality and tastes better than milk put through ordinary pasteurization. Under this system, the milk is not homogenized, separated, or standardized. Handling the milk as little as possible safeguards more of the milk's nutritional value and cream content, as well as its farm-fresh flavor. Many small family dairies such as California's Strauss Family Creamery, Ohio's Hartzler's Family Dairy, and Iowa's Kalona Organics now sell vat-pasteurized milk. Whole Foods now sells a variety of vat pasteurized dairy products. Now that you have all the information on vat and ordinary pasteurized and homogenized milk, you can make your own decision about which version you prefer. If I were a milk drinker, I would go for raw milk as my first choice and any other type of low-fat milk as a second choice. My reasoning is that if I'm not consuming raw milk with all its amazing nutritional value then I would opt for a lower fat version of milk because at that point it's about weight control benefits. It's that simple.

A Word about Soy

Soy has been eaten in Asia since around 2000 BC and is traditionally served in a fermented form that has shown to be quite healthful for traditional Asian cultures. American culture has been in existence for less than 400 years. Soy, as it is used here and now, is often farmed with chemicals and processed into odd shapes and colors to resemble all sorts of dubious food items (for example, hot dogs). Then people eat these processed things and are subsequently shocked to discover that there are health consequences.

Research has shown that consuming excessive amounts of soy causes endocrine disruption and digestive problems and can be associated with thyroid problems, fertility issues, and problems with sex drive. Some studies have shown that it even has the potential to contribute to certain cancers. What makes the soy issue so confusing is that for every study that proves a connection between soy and reduced disease risk there is another study that challenges these claims. The fact is soy is a $4 billion industry in the U.S., and the soy industry is a major backer of studies that have proven the benefits of eating soy. For its part, besides promoting heart health, the industry claims soy can alleviate symptoms associated with menopause; reduce the risk of certain cancers, and lower levels of the "bad" cholesterol. So what is the answer?

My feeling is that eating traditional Asian soy products, farmed without toxic chemicals, is probably just fine. Soy foods such as tofu, tempeh, and miso have been part of the diet in Asian countries for centuries and are only minimally processed.

Here are a few soy food brands rated highly on the Soy Scorecard of the Cornucopia Institute (an objective, independent research and advocacy organization). Personally, I love Silk Organic Soymilk because it's made with organic non-GMO soybeans and it tastes fantastic.

SOY MILK	OTHER SOY PRODUCTS
Eden Foods	Rhapsody Natural Foods
Tofu Shop	Unisoya
Twin Oaks	Small Planet
Vermont Soy	Farm Soy
	Green Cuisine

Milk Alternatives: Got Not-Milk?

For folks who choose to steer clear of dairy milk for whatever reason—perhaps they're lactose intolerant or they live a vegan lifestyle, or maybe they just don't like milk—there are a number of alternatives on the market today. Here's the down-low on these alternatives.

Almond Milk

The Perks It's really low in calories and fat (approximately 50 calories, 2.5 grams fat, and 8 grams carbs per cup). Like almonds, it's rich in the antioxidant vitamin E, protein, and omega-3 fat. It also contains other minerals like zinc, iron, magnesium, and calcium. What it doesn't have is the all the controversy that comes with soy milk. That's because it's basically made up of ground almonds and water.

Drawbacks As a result of the high cost of almonds, there may not be enough almonds in many brands of almond milk to have enough of the minerals listed above. Read the side of your almond milk carton and you may find that almonds are the second or third ingredient following water and sweeteners. Therefore, look for almond milk that has almonds at the top of the ingredient list and that doesn't have added sweeteners. In addition, most almonds are sprayed with several pesticides, so opt for organic almond milk whenever possible.

Coconut Milk

The Perks My personal favorite of all the milk options. I use this every day in my tea and smoothies. Coconut milk sold both in cartons and by the can is amazing. (Canned coconut milk is just coconut and water—talk about a *real food!*) It's lighter, sweeter, and is a delicious substitute for cow's milk in cereal and coffee and for cooking. Loaded with nutrients, coconut milk has 50 percent of your recommended daily allowance of vitamin B_{12}, 30 percent of vitamin D, and 10 percent of both magnesium and calcium. You may have heard it's really high in saturated fats, but those fats are actually medium chain fatty acids, a good fat. Specifically, one of the fats is lauric acid, which is known to build the immune system in a big way. I believe it's the best milk substitute available, and since I'm lactose intolerant it's what I drink.

Drawbacks The taste is sweet, so it doesn't work in many savory recipes; it's better in dessert recipes or smoothies. It's also not a very good source of protein in the way that cow's milk is. And read the ingredients, because some brands have less than desirable additives like sugar, food coloring, and preservatives. My favorite coconut milk brands are Thai Kitchen, A Taste of Thai, Trader Joe's, and So Delicious. Both regular and light coconut milk are good for the real-food diet. I'm personally a huge coconut milk fan; in my opinion, the nutritional and weight loss benefits outweigh these few drawbacks.

Soy Milk

The Perks Soy milk is fortified with Vitamin D as is cow's milk. One cup has 35 percent of your recommended daily allowance of vitamin D and 6 grams of protein.

Drawbacks Soy milk is shrouded with controversy, much of it stemming from the fact that the phytoestrogens found in soy function similar to the way estrogen does. There is evidence that these phytoestrogens can cause an increased risk of breast cancer as well as some issues with infertility. However, the research is ongoing and nothing is written in stone. My advice is that if you want to drink soy milk, do it in moderation, and seek out the brands listed on page 138 to make sure you're getting the least factory-processed product.

Rice Milk

The Perks Fortified rice milk contains vitamins A and D.
Drawbacks It's a refined carb; stay away from it.

Canned and Frozen Foods: A Surprising Benefit

Canned and frozen foods may possibly come with fewer pesticides, although most of the research has been done by the food industry. The washing and blanching to prepare fruits and vegetables for canning or freezing removes or destroys approximately 80 percent to 90 percent of pesticide residues, according to the U.S.-based National Food Processors Association.

Canned Foods: The BPA Controversy

My experience with canned goods goes back to when I first got my driver's license and my grandmother would have me drive her to what she referred to as "the canned goods store." Grandma loved to go there and buy cases of canned tomato sauce, tomato paste, stewed tomatoes, string beans, corn, and peas; the cans were bashed-in and therefore available for pennies on the dollar. Although we had a ranch that provided all of the above, she couldn't resist a sale. Anyway, if Grandma knew that those canned goods had a chemical in them that could possibly be harmful to our health—bisphenol A (BPA)—she would be peeved!

What is BPA? Bisphenol A is a chemical found in cans and the hard plastics in baby bottles and other plastic food containers. Because they may leach into food, there is a growing concern about their effects on humans. In some animal studies, researchers have noted that BPA causes developmental changes, but it's not clear what harm, if any, it may cause to humans.

Taking this into consideration, I don't feel that we need to avoid all canned foods. Rather, as consumers, we need to nudge food and plastic manufacturers to phase out their use of BPA in their products. The good news is that some manufactures are several steps ahead of the game and offer BPA-free products.

Each of the following companies has started using BPA-free can linings for certain products, is committed to removing the chemical from all of its packaging products, and has a time line by which to achieve this transition.

Eden Foods has been leading the BPA-free way for years, with a policy in place since 1999, and packages all of its organic bean products in cans lined without BPA.

Hain Celestial's brands include Health Valley, Earth's Best, and Westbrae Natural.

ConAgra owns brands such as Chef Boyardee, Hunt's, and Healthy Choice.

H.J. Heinz and the three companies above received the highest scores in this report.

Trader Joe's has gone BPA-free for some products, including canned corn and beans and some meat products.

Real-Foodie Kristen Michaelis

Kristen Michaelis grew up eating a typical "healthy" American factory food diet. Instead of sugary cereal, she ate Shredded Wheat and Raisin Bran; instead of white bread, wheat bread was served. However, like the majority of us, fish was cooked in factory vegetable oils, Crisco was in the cupboard, margarine was in the fridge, and refined carbs were the norm.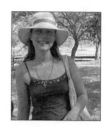

After she gave birth to her first son, a friend came by with the documentary *The Future of Food*, and that was her catalyst for beginning her real-food journey. "That was the first time I ever thought of food in terms of the environment, and our health," she recalls. "It was the first time I realized there was more to the story than meets the eye when you go into the grocery store. Before that, if the packet said it was healthy, then I believed it was, end of story."

After watching *The Future of Food*, Kristen set about educating herself on where her food comes from. She also joined a CSA, a community supported agricultural program, and made friends with other folks interested in living a real-food lifestyle. "I started taking baby steps more and more into what I consider traditional real food," she said. That was 6 years ago. Today, Kristen has transformed her eating habits and is living the life of a real-food renegade. In fact, that's the name of her insanely inspiring blog, www.foodrenegade.com. Her blog is a feast of real-food recipes, nutrition, and health articles, and gives us the latest in what's going on in sustainable agriculture, food politics, and food philosophy.

I had an amazing conversation with Kristen, who was generous enough to share her wealth of knowledge with me as well as one of her favorite recipes! Check out our chat, starting on the next page, and don't miss the fantastic versatile broccoli recipe she was gracious enough to share with us!

What advice do you give folks who are just starting out on their real-food journey?

I tell people there are two things you can change: one is to prioritize your food choices in ways that are going to make the biggest impact on your health; and the second is to change the way you manage your kitchen.

There are a lot of things that you can do. For example, people think that cooking everything from scratch or mostly from scratch takes tons more time than a convenience meal, but I've seen studies that show differently. A person cooking from scratch can still get a cooked meal to the table in 30 minutes just like the person doing the convenience cooking. The biggest difference is in the actual prep time. When you're preparing a meal from scratch, the time you spend in the kitchen, you're actually doing something in the kitchen to get the meal on the table. When you're doing the convenience food meal thing, you pop something in the microwave or the oven, and while it's cooking you do something else in your house. So it's a little bit more work, but it still takes the same amount of time to put the food on the table. So I would start by encouraging people to eliminate packaged and processed food and start cooking things from scratch. And by the way, for those who believe it's more expensive to eat real food, you can actually save money.

For instance, you can save up and buy things in bulk. That reduces the cost significantly. For example, if you shop at a farmers' market, there is always a week where all of the farmers have a super over-abundance of a certain food item. If that week you decide to buy two buckets of strawberries for a great price, you can freeze them, and you've got frozen strawberries to hold you through the summer that are locally grown and organic and you've paid a cheaper price.

Or people don't realize how many meals you can get if you buy a whole chicken. You can easily make three or four meals out of a good-sized whole chicken. [For instance, you can eat the roasted chicken the first night, make chicken salad with the leftovers, or chicken enchiladas, and then boil the carcass for chicken broth afterwards that can be used to cook up countless different soups.]

You're such a fantastic blogger, your outreach, how you're helping others. How important is it to access blogs and become a part of the real-food community? Do you think it's important to be part of a community of like-minded people who can support you?

Unfortunately, for some folks who switch to real food, they might not get support from family members or friends. In that case, you need to go online because any time you make changes like this you need support and you need to know that you're not crazy. It's also a great way to get ideas and motivation to sustain any kind of change without that kind of support. That is where the bloggers and other real-food-inspired Web sites are a real help.

If I looked in your pantry right now, what oils would I find?

I have a giant container of coconut oil and other traditional nut oils, such as macadamia nut oil. You actually can cook with macadamia nut oil, it has a really nice nut taste, but it tends to be expensive so you probably wouldn't want to.

What is one of your favorite recipes?

One of my family's favorite comfort foods is a steamy plate of cheesy versatile broccoli casserole. Of course, the version I grew up eating was made with Cheez Whiz (seriously). As an adult, I adapted it into a main course by adding cut up chunks of sausage. Then, as a real-foodie, I adapted it further by creating my own easy cheese sauce. Lately, as a low-carber, I've been adapting it even further by cutting out the rice and using grated cauliflower.

I'm going to let you guys in on how to make it—with meat or no meat, rice or cauliflower. After all, it's the cheesy broccoli part that truly makes the dish. and, I'm going to let you in on how to make it in a single skillet, no hot oven necessary.

Kristen's Cheesy Broccoli Casserole

2 tablespoons butter

1 head of broccoli, chopped

1 small onion, chopped

4 cups cooked brown rice (or grated cauliflower)

1 pound cooked meat (nitrate-free sausage is my favorite, or you could go meatless)

4 tablespoons flour

1 cup milk (from grass fed cows)

8 ounces grated cheese (experiment! I love a sharp cheddar, but I've made it with smoked gouda, too)

½ cup sour cream

Salt and pepper to taste

In a large (12-inch), deep skillet, melt 2 tablespoons of the butter and add the broccoli, onions, and cauliflower (if not using rice). Cook over medium heat, occasionally stirring, until veggies are tender. Add cooked meat (if using) and cooked rice (if using).

Scoot the cooked vegetable medley off to the edges of the skillet, creating a well in the middle, just over the burner. Reduce heat to medium-low. Melt the remaining 2 tablespoons of butter in the well, then quickly stir in flour to make a hot roux. When the roux is mixed and bubbly, pour in cold milk and continue stirring, raising heat to medium. As the mixture thickens, begin stirring the vegetables into the sauce.

Evenly distribute the cheese over the whole skillet, and continue stirring the contents. Once cheese is melted, remove the casserole from heat. Stir in sour cream, and add salt and pepper to taste.

I feel confident that, armed with the guidance from this chapter, you're ready to tackle the supermarket. But, hey, why go if you don't have to? In the next chapter, I'll show you avenues you can take so that you can spend less time in the supermarket and more time making friends and enjoying the sunshine.

CHAPTER 10

Get Out of the Supermarket

In the last chapter, I took you through the supermarket for guidance on how to get real food into your shopping basket. In this chapter, I'm taking you out of the supermarket to show you the many opportunities available to get *the* most *uh-mazing* locally grown and raised real food. Some of them, like farmers' markets, you're probably familiar with, but others, like food swaps and www.foodzie.com, a totally fab online farmers' market, you might not be aware of. So, in this chapter, I take you on a tour of some of the best ways to find real food for you and your fam without setting foot in a supermarket. So grab your recyclable bags, and away we go!

A Trip to the Farmers' Market

In the past decade, the number of farmers' markets has exploded across the country. There are now more than 6,000 nationwide, and 900 of them are open during winter. That's about a 250 percent increase since 1994. (Your local farmers' market is hands down *the* best place to buy fresh, locally grown food—food that's not a product of the processed food industry. I guarantee that the fresh produce, the just-laid eggs, the pasture-raised beef, poultry, and pork, the jars of honey, the fresh baked bread—whatever you buy at the farmers' market—will taste better than anything you could buy at the supermarket.

Farmers' markets have blossomed in more ways than just in numbers since the onset of the real-food movement. Not only do they offer a way for us to connect with the source of our food, they also provide us with a place to nurture community and celebrate local food cultures. Each farmers' market has a different vibe and personality. Like heirloom tomatoes, no two are the same. Typically, in addition to the produce you would expect, a wide variety of other products are available, including eggs, milk, cream, ice cream, butter, cheese, honey, maple syrup, jams, jellies, sauces, mushrooms, nuts, flowers, free range poultry, and pasture-raised beef, pork, lamb, and goat, plus wool, wine, olive oil, vinegar, fresh bread, pies, pickles, and pastries. Prepared items are increasing in prevalence at today's farmers' markets, which is great for all of us busy folks.

Another trend is the presence of your favorite farmers' markets and their vendors on Facebook and Twitter. How fun is that?! For example, Oregon's Portland Farmers Market tweets about its various contests, like offering $100 to whoever tweets back the best use of a pear. And most have great Web sites and blogs. In addition, many are now offering classes to customers, such as preserving classes or kids' cooking classes. Fantastic!

While in many ways these aren't your grandpa's farmers' markets, shopping at them is like taking a step back into the past—in such a good way—a time before the industrial food frenzy took hold of our food distribution system. Think about it: Farmers' markets are a traditional way of selling agricultural and homemade products. (I love the word "homemade.") In addition to the feeling of carrying on an important tradition, there's a lot else to feel good about when shopping at a farmers' market. For one thing, you're helping local farms stay in business. For another, you're helping conserve natural resources. That's because, according to the American Farmland Trust, sustainably managed farms conserve soil and clean water and provide a habitat for wildlife.

Now that I've given you the DL on what's going on in the farmers' market world, I want to break it down a bit. Because it's a totally different experience from shopping in a supermarket, here are a few tried and true farmers' market shopping tips.

Farmers' Market Tips and Tricks

1. Ask the vendors questions. Some I ask are:

    -   Is this type of produce in season here?
    -   Where exactly was it grown?
    -   How was it grown? With this question, you're looking to understand if any fertilizer, pesticides, or herbicides were used. Also, it's useful to know if the produce was grown in a polyculture (many different plant species) field or as part of a large monoculture. Also, while you're at it, ask if the farmer grows any plants that are GMOs.
    -   What do you feed your animals? (Note: Farmers' markets are a great place to find pasture-raised meat and free range chicken; you might pay a bit more for poultry and meat raised this way, but the trick is to cut down on the amount of protein you get from animals in the first place. By doing this, you can afford to buy the good stuff when you do eat it.)

2. Bring cash! Sometimes there's an ATM set up, but not always, and many vendors accept only cash.

3. Make a list and have a plan. Once you're familiar with the setup of your farmers' market, and knowing what's in season and when is old hat, it will be easier to plan what you're going to buy for your week of eating. Since there's never a guarantee that they'll have exactly what you want, have a Plan A and a Plan B. Don't be totally rigid about what you buy! Feel free to explore and try new things, and to be inspired by the ingredients to cook new dishes. Just also make sure you don't come home with a bunch of interesting new produce and ingredients you've never heard of, and have nothing to eat for the week because you didn't get your staples and you have no idea what to do with your motley crew

of items. You can start with a general plan, like "lettuce for salad," " veggies for a salad," "fruit for breakfast and to snack on," "veggies for a pasta dish"—you get the idea. Then if you see something you want to try or that inspires you to look up a new recipe online, go for it! After all, kohlrabi and cardoons are what happen while you're making other plans!

4. Bring your own bags. Get with the program, and be on your best environmentally friendly behavior at the farmers' market. Walking around with plastic bags is one surefire way to be branded a newbie!

5. Have a few flexible recipes in your cooking repertoire so that you can just fill in the blanks with whatever you happen to find that day at the market. If you see a bunch of amazing veggies you're not familiar with, you can have a go-to recipe to get you warmed up cooking them for the first time. See Chapter 12 for a few of my favorites, one of which I borrowed from real-foodie Lisa Leake, who is a fabulous cook!

That's Ripe!

While shopping for produce at the farmers' market, you'll notice that some fruits and veggies are more ripe or not as fresh as others. Here are a few tips for picking out vegetables:

Arugula: Go for unblemished, springy, deep-colored leaves. Arugula is relatively fragile and perishable, so either use it within a couple of days of buying it or extend its shelf life by sticking its stem end in a glass of water and covering the whole thing with a plastic bag.

Avocado: If that little brown nubbin of stem falls off with a slight touch, it's ready to buy. Also, if it's ready to eat, it will give at the touch when you press on it. If you can only eat half at a time, refrigerate the unused half with the pit still in. Just squeeze some lemon juice on it, wrap it tight in plastic wrap, and refrigerate.

Cantaloupe: Look at the webbing on the cantaloupe. If it's wide, that means the cantaloupe is ripe and sweet. However, it must also be firm, without bruising or soft spots.

Cauliflower: Cauliflower will last longer if you choose one that is firm and has no space between the floret heads. The leaves should be fresh and green. Avoid buying cauliflower that has small dark brown spots. It is a sign of spoilage and will not last long.

Cucumbers: Avoid cucumbers that are soft, yellowish, or wrinkled on the ends. A good cucumber has an even dark green color, and is firm and relatively thin. A good cucumber can be either long or short, but big fat cucumbers tend to be full of seeds and can taste bitter. As a result, it is actually better to choose slender cucumbers instead of larger ones. I have found that Persian cucumbers are consistently the best tasting and have just the right amount of crispiness.

Green beans: Bend one; if it's fresh it will snap into two pieces.

Eggplant, Squash, Zucchini: Avoid buying soft or wrinkled squash, zucchini, or eggplant. The firmer the vegetable, the longer it will last in your refrigerator.

Fennel: When you're buying fennel, look for smooth, white, densely packed bulbs.

Kiwi: Look for kiwis that are very firm; they will keep in the refrigerator for months. If you want the kiwi to ripen fast, take it out of the refrigerator and let it ripen at room temperature.

Ready to Go?

Now it's time for you to find a local farmers' market in your area. The easiest place to search is at www.localharvest.org. Go to the home page, search for "farmers' markets" and your zip code or city. You can also go to http://apps.ams.usda.gov/FarmersMarkets/, type in your state and voilà—a list of farmers' markets near you!

Merry Chri . . . uh, CSA Box Delivery!

Another great way to stay out of the supermarket is to invest in a CSA, or Community Supported Agriculture—a partnership between a local farmer or groups of farmers and consumers. Basically, you pay so much a month, maybe $30, and each week you'll receive a box of fresh veggies—whatever's ready for sale from the farm. It's kind of like being a shareholder in the crop and each week getting paid your dividend in veggies. Belonging to a CSA is like having Christmas every week. You'll look forward to opening up your box and seeing what's inside. Growers often throw in a *lagniappe* (a little something extra; pronounced "lan-YAP"), like a loaf of fresh bread or some preserves. Within the last 10 years, CSAs have become more popular as the buy-local movement has exploded. It's now pretty easy to find a CSA, whether you live in New York City or in the hill country of Texas. Again, www.localharvest.org is the best place to find a CSA near you. Here are a few things to consider if you're thinking about joining a CSA:

Cost: CSA shares typically cost from $400 to $600 for the entire season, which breaks down to about $20 to $30 a week for 20 weeks. Some CSAs offer worker shares: free vegetables if you work one day a week on the farm or reduced costs if you work one or two shifts per growing season. As a less costly option, some CSAs offer half shares, which are smaller boxes every week or a box every other week. This is a great option because a typical box of veggies in the heart of the growing season can be extremely bountiful and might be much more than your family can eat in a week's time. (This is the option I use with my CSA.) Yet another option is to split a share with a friend or neighbor.

A box full of ???: In addition to the standard tomatoes, apples, lettuce, bell peppers, and so on, you'll get introduced to some unfamiliar produce. That's part of the fun. But if you don't like surprises, discuss this with the farmer and see if you can have more of a say in what's dropped in your box.

The pickup: You'll want to find a CSA with a pickup location that's convenient for you. Most make it easy, and will have the box ready for you at their table at a farmers' market near you. Each week you can pick up a new box and drop off your empty one.

Extra bonus: Some CSAs offer fruit, dairy, egg, meat, bread, or even fish shares.

Local Harvest: The Real-food Yellow Pages

In order to eat real food, you have to know where to find it near where you live, and on top of that you need to know where to get it when you're traveling or if you've relocated. So thank goodness there's www .localharvest.org. The Web site is basically a real-food directory; I like to think of it as the real-food Yellow Pages. (For all you younger folks, that's a telephone book that lists businesses.) LocalHarvest maintains an up-to-date, definitive, reliable nationwide public directory of small farms, farmers' markets, CSAs, co-ops, natural groceries, restaurants, and farms. The LocalHarvest search engine helps us find products from family farms and local sources of sustainably grown food, and encourages us to reach out and make contact with small farms in our area. Plus, LocalHarvest has an online store where small farmers can sell their wares. LocalHarvest operates under the philosophy that the best food is the food that's grown and raised closest to you. So if you're looking to find a farm where you can buy grass fed beef or orange blossom honey or free range duck eggs, all you have to do is log on to www .localharvest.org.

Where to Buy Free Range and Grass Fed Meat Online

Eatwild.com: An excellent resource that will help you find local farmers that have embraced the practices of grass fed, free range, organic, and humane farming.

U.S. Wellness Meats: If you wish to have your meat delivered to your doorstep, this is an excellent place to order from online. Just go to the site, www.grasslandbeef.com, and click on the Protocol link to read about how it raises its livestock.

Blackwing Quality Meats: Another great source of free range poultry and grass fed meat (www.blackwing.com).

Real-Foodie Nina Planck

Nina Planck is a farmer's daughter, food writer, farmers' market entrepreneur, local-foodist, and advocate for traditional foods. Nina is one of the most well-known, well-respected real-food advocates in the U.S. After reading Nina's work, you'll be liberated to eat all the real foods your ancestors ate, such as red meat, butter, and lard. Her books include *The Farmers' Market Cookbook, Real Food: What to Eat and Why*, and *Real Food for Mother and Baby,* and she's the founder of the wildly popular London Farmers' Markets. I asked Nina about food. Here's what she had to say.

What foods did you grow up eating?

My mother raised us on real food, plain old American-style. Meat, vegetables, whole grains, real milk, and cheese. We made our own bread and granola. We had desserts, but not often, and only real desserts with good ingredients and never, ever, too much sugar. My mother used to say, "No matter how poor we are, we'll always have real butter, olive oil, and maple syrup."

What advice would you give about the natural sugars being sold in natural food stores today, such as unrefined sugars, organic cane sugar, organic dehydrated cane sugar, Sucanat, and Raw Sugar?

All sugars are really an industrial food in the quantity we eat them now. Even a thin man shouldn't have too much honey or maple syrup. We should eat these things in moderation. I mean sparingly. That said, there is a small difference traditionally between the worst forms of sugar and the best natural sweeteners. Alas, they all contribute to high and low blood sugar, weight gain, and obesity. However, there is no substitute for plain white sugar, so I buy the best organic and whole I can find when I want pure sweetener because lemon meringue pie just does not taste good if made with maple syrup. Same story with dark chocolate and raspberry jam. You have to consider the place sweets have in your diet. Too much dessert is simply not good for your body. Nearly anything that is true of sugar is true of all the sweeteners.

What do you think of the healthier versions of processed foods, such as the all-natural versions of saltines, chocolate chip cookies, graham crackers, even cinnamon rolls? What would your advice be, because some people think "If I get it from Whole Foods, it's okay"?

The only improvement on these foods and diet ingredients is the agricultural improvement. Organic agriculture is clearly better than industrial agriculture, but don't fool yourself, processed foods are still heavily processed, they're still not fresh, and they're often broken foods; that is, they take a whole food, break it down, and then they reassemble it to look and taste a certain way. The best foods in the supermarket still come from the outer aisles. But you do have to visit the middle aisles to get the olive oil and brown rice.

What do you think of Walmart's efforts to make real foods more affordable to folks?

I think its great news. I think it's great when a huge retailer adds an organic line, bans trans fats, or stops using some artificial ingredients. It's a step forward. Sometimes it's a giant step forward and sometimes it's a small step.

In your book you mentioned that you lost weight after you started eating a real-food diet. How exactly would you explain this?

I was a low-fat, fat-free vegetarian and I ate a lot of fruits and vegetables, fat-free foods like yogurt, and a whole lot of carbohydrates. I was missing fats and proteins. Fats and proteins are an essential part of being at a healthy weight. In fact I wouldn't be surprised if I didn't eat more calories now at 125 pounds than I did as a fat-free carbohydrate-eating vegetarian weighing 145 pounds. I do not, and do not recommend, counting calories or grams or micrograms of anything. It doesn't help you eat.

What kind of butter do you like?

We like any good butter. There are good French, English, and Irish butters. There are some good American butters such as Straus Creamery in California and Kate's from Maine. Organic Pastures makes a really good butter, and it has a delicious sea-sonal butter from pasture raised cows. You can freeze it if you want it year-round.

What do you think are some of the more exciting developments in the real-food market?

Convenience foods and frozen foods. One of our local farmers is now selling frozen corn off the cob. I love it. I use a lot of tomato sauce, and I'm so glad it can now be local. I love basic, local, preserved, real seasonal convenience foods partly because I'm now a mother of three children and I depend on it. People love and need convenience food, and that is the proper way to do it.

CHAPTER 11

Real-Food Weight Loss in Action

You are now armed with all the information you need to go out into the world and gather real food. As I mentioned in Chapter 6, if you make the switch to a real-food diet, you *will* lose weight. But to really maximize your weight loss, you'll want to follow the real-food weight loss guidelines I introduced in that chapter. In this chapter, I'll show you how to use the various tools you've learned throughout the book to make the different components of the diet work in your everyday life. First, you'll create your own Real-Food Charter to guide your food choices. Then I'll walk you through all the elements of the real-food diet and show you how they work in real life. In addition, I give you the down-low on a host of amazing real-food weight loss ingredients, like coconut and fermented foods that fit in fantastically with my real-food weight loss plan. Most helpful of all, this chapter includes 2 weeks of delicious meal plans for the real-food weight loss diet. Plus, a bonus meal plan for anyone who wants to jump on the fast track for weight loss.

Your Real-Food Charter
and an 80/20 or 90/10 Option

Now that you've been given the information you need to separate the real from the fake, it's time for you to sit down and pen your personal Real-Food Charter. Before you do, I'd first like to stress that you should view your charter as "living," and by that I mean that it's a set of personal, informed dietary guidelines that you reserve the right to change as you see fit over time as you change and evolve during your real-food journey. To help you get your charter organized, I suggest that you divide it into a few different categories, such as "meat," "dairy," and so on. Then, within the categories (where applicable), include spaces for "if possible" and "second best choice" options. In addition, include a category for the ingredients and foods that will have no place on your real-food table and a category for an explanation of the exceptions you will make. Take a look at this sample charter to get the idea.

MY REAL-FOOD CHARTER

MEAT

If possible:
Second choice:

PRODUCE

If possible:
Second choice:

DAIRY

If possible:
Second choice:

BREAD

COOKING OILS AND FATS

BEVERAGES

COMPLETELY OFF THE TABLE

EXCEPTIONS

Speaking of exceptions, one thing I would like to make clear is that many real-foodies, including myself, live a more or less 80/20 or 90/10 real-food lifestyle. In our culture, it's nearly impossible to completely steer clear of things like refined carbs (they're in chocolate, for goodness sake, and a life without chocolate wouldn't seem real to me!) or factory oils and so on. Plus, you want to enjoy your life with your family and friends. If you're at a family member's wedding, do you really think turning down a piece of wedding cake is the way to live? I don't. As long as you eat a healthy, real-food diet the majority of the time, then you're in good shape. Having said that, weight loss is a whole different deal. The closer to 100 percent real foods in your diet, the better your chances of losing weight. This chapter is designed to help you achieve weight loss through a real-food diet in the real world. Read on.

The Real-Food Weight Loss Diet

As you'll recall from Chapter 6, consuming real food leads to weight loss because of the nutrients that are added to the diet—fiber and omega-3 fats—and the ingredients that are removed from the diet—added sugar, all other refined carbs, refined salt, and harmful additives and preservatives. Applying the correct balance to the diet—eating the optimal mix of nutrients at regular intervals—guarantees that weight loss will be one outcome of adopting a real-food diet. In sum, there are three simple rules to the real-food diet:

1. Eat a **PC** (protein-carb) or **FC** (fat-carb) combo every **4 hours**

2. Avoid anything **refined** (sugars, carbohydrates, salts) and **harmful** additives and preservatives

3. Consume **fiber** and **omega-3 fatty acids** every day

In Parts I and II, I spend a lot of time discussing the harmful ingredients mentioned in rule #2. Remember that refined sugar, carbs, and salt all contribute to overeating. As for steering clear of harmful additives and preservatives, at least one of the most common—MSG—has been found to contribute to weight gain. This is a relatively recent finding, and it makes me wonder about the possibility that other additives also interfere with weight loss. In addition, research has shown that harmful additives and preservatives compromise health. To set yourself up for the utmost success in losing weight, you want to be your strongest, healthiest self, so I've given you lots of tools to help you get off the stuff.

Now that you know how to identify and get rid of the fake foods, in this section I discuss how you can incorporate rules #1 and #3, adding real foods with real nutrients into your weight-loss plan.

Do a Protein-Carb-Fat Balancing Act at Every Meal

One important strategy when it comes to losing weight is to balance proteins, carbs, and fats at every meal. *Basically, you always want to make sure you're pairing your carbs with either protein or fat.* And remember to choose complex carbs like vegetables, fruits, and whole grains. Doing this leads to balanced blood sugar levels, and balanced blood sugar levels put the brakes on maddening food cravings and nagging hunger.

The ideal meal will be a PCF (protein-carb-fat) combo; that is, it will contain all three macronutrients. This is rule number one for anyone following this real-food diet. For instance, try a dinner of a grass fed rib eye, baked sweet potato, and grilled veggies. You're getting fat and protein from the rib eye and complex carbs from the sweet potato and grilled veggies. If you'd like to throw a side salad dressed with olive oil and vinegar into the mix, that's fine too. The veggies add more complex carbs and the olive oil, some good fat.

As a general rule, aim to get approximately 20 percent of your calories from protein, 50 percent from complex carbs, and the remaining 30 percent from real fats. But I don't want you to be focused on counting calories. A good rule of thumb is to make sure veggies are taking up half of your plate; protein should be about the size of a deck of cards if it's meat, or take up a third of your plate if it's not meat; fat should be kept to a minimum. I stress eating only real fats (organic butter, walnuts, coconut oil, and olive oil), not only because they have myriad health benefits but also because they all aid in weight loss (plus, most of them contain omega-3 fatty acids).

You may be wondering why the rule is not to eat a PCF combo every 4 hours. I notice that my nutrition clients do not have to work to add fat to meals. Fat gets into our meals without very much effort at all, whereas finding unrefined carbohydrates and healthy protein sources can be a bit more challenging. So it's better for you to work toward combining a real-food protein with a real-food carb, because the fat will automatically fall into place. Also, at some meals, you may not be able to fit in all three macronutrients. In that case, opt for a PC (protein-carb) or FC (fat-carb) combo. For instance, if you eat a slice of toast for breakfast, spread a thin layer of real butter on it. I know this sounds counterintuitive, but the butter helps slow down the digestion of the toast and keeps you feeling full longer.

Reach for Real Food Every 4 Hours

Eating every 4 hours is a great way to keep blood sugar levels balanced and avoid food cravings. Plus, it helps speed up your metabolism, causing you to burn pounds faster. Just make sure you're eating controlled portions. Your schedule will dictate how this particular balancing act plays out in your own personal situation. Here is a simple breakdown of one way to pull off eating every 4 hours.

Let's say you wake up at 6 a.m. Here is what your schedule would look like.

6:00 a.m.	Wake
7:00 a.m.	Meal #1
11:00 a.m.	Meal #2
3:00 p.m.	Meal #3
7:00 p.m.	Meal #4

Okay, so I bet you are saying to yourself . . . but what if I can't eat my lunch at 11 a.m.? No worries, here is the deal: You have the option to eat an entire meal if you are hungry and have the time to do so. If you are not able to eat a complete meal, your best bet is to keep a small snack with you. For example, you could snack on walnuts and dried fruit, or cheese and fresh fruit (like string cheese and an orange). These are all foods you can easily keep handy in your purse, briefcase, desk, or backpack (and yes, it's okay if string cheese is unrefrigerated for a couple of hours). This will keep your blood sugar levels stable and metabolism humming.

What if your meal plan is to eat dinner at 7:00 p.m., but you have a dinner engagement at 8:30? Try eating about half a meal at 7 and half of a normal portion of whatever is served at the dinner event. After that, your next meal should be about 4 hours later (if you are still awake and hungry; otherwise, just go to sleep).

In the real world of eating and real food, timing may not always be perfect. . . . So if you end up eating too early or too late, don't stress out. Just be mindful that it is best to wait 4 hours between meals—but not too much longer—for optimal weight loss, and do your best to make that happen. If weight loss is your goal, I am confident you will find a way to carve your schedule to make it work for you. If my clients at Passages in Malibu can pull it off as they are going through rehab, you can too. Where there is a will, there is always a way.

Adding Fiber

An important part of making the switch is increasing the amount of vegetables, whole grains, beans, and fruits you eat, making them the foundation of your real-food diet. One of the best perks you'll get from incorporating them into your everyday diet is that these are the foods that are chock full of fiber. Because fiber keeps you feeling full longer, you won't be tempted to overeat. Some of the best sources of fiber are

EXCELLENT SOURCES OF FIBER (5 OR MORE GRAMS PER SERVING)

- Barley
- Black beans
- Buckwheat
- Fennel
- Grapefruit
- Lentils

- Lima beans
- Navy beans
- Oats
- Pinto beans
- Split peas
- Swiss chard

VERY GOOD SOURCES OF FIBER (1.5 OR MORE GRAMS PER SERVING)

- Apricots
- Beets
- Cranberries
- Eggplant
- Flaxseeds

- Green beans
- Shiitake mushrooms
- Strawberries
- Sweet potato

GOOD SOURCES OF FIBER (0.5 GRAM OR MORE PER SERVING)

- Broccoli
- Cauliflower
- Celery
- Collard greens

- Mustard greens
- Romaine lettuce
- Spinach
- Turnip greens

Omega-3s

As you recall from Chapter 6, omega-3s, such as those found in fish, prevent obesity and help with weight loss by regulating blood sugar levels and burning fat.

In general, you should make sure you're getting at least one source of omega-3s a day. Seafood is one of the very best sources of omega-3s. One way to make sure you're getting enough omega-3 in your diet in general is to eat seafood twice a week. *Tip: A good way to do this is to make one of your lunches a tuna fish sandwich on whole wheat bread or a whole wheat wrap and to serve seafood for one of your weeknight or weekend dinners.*

Other ways to stock up on omega-3s are to eat one or more of the following omega-3 laden foods a day:

OTHER EXCELLENT SOURCES OF OMEGA-3S

- Flaxseed oil
- Flaxseeds: Be sure to buy ground flaxseeds, because your body can't access the nutrients when the seed is whole. *Tip: Ground flaxseeds are great in oatmeal and in smoothies.*
- Walnuts

VERY GOOD SOURCES OF OMEGA-3S

- Chia seeds: *Tip: Chia seeds are great in oatmeal and smoothies.*
- Raw tofu

VEGETABLE AND FRUIT SOURCES THAT HAVE A BIT OF OMEGA-3

- Broccoli
- Brussels sprouts
- Cabbage
- Cauliflower
- Collard greens
- Green beans
- Kale
- Miso

- Olive oil
- Pumpkin seeds
- Raspberries
- Soy beans
- Strawberries
- Summer squash
- Turnip greens
- Winter squash

Additional Real-Food Weight Loss Tools

If all you do is follow the three real-food diet rules I've given you, I promise you'll see the pounds start to melt away. But if you're truly motivated, there are some additional things you can do and foods you can try that will boost your results and make it easier to stick to the rules.

PRACTICE PORTION CONTROL

Here in the U.S. we are used to oversize portions. Part of eating a real-food diet is eating real portions, meaning that you eat the amount of food you need to feel satisfied, rather than stuffed. It's not necessary to count calories or grams of proteins, carbs, and fat on the real-food weight loss diet. Rather, the goal is to learn to focus on shopping, preparing, and eating real food as often as possible. If you just focus on eating real food, *weight loss will follow.*

Part of the reason is that the two major nutrients you're adding when you eat read food—fiber and omega-3 fats—both have the effect of making you feel full. So, while you might be able to eat a whole plate of pasta (a refined carb) without feeling satisfied, you may find that you can't eat more than half a plate of quinoa with kale, cranberries, and walnuts.

However, when you're just starting out, you might continue to load your plate simply out of force of habit. Bear in mind that anything in excess is a bad thing, and that goes for real food. Just because something is considered a real food doesn't give you license to eat as much of it as you want. Although I don't want you to get bogged down actually counting the calories, remember that everything you eat does have calories. So here are a few general rules to help you learn what real portions look like.

- **Meat/protein:** A serving of meat should be no bigger than the size of your palm (about 20 to 25 grams per meal or 10 to 15 grams per snack).

- **Carbs:** A serving of carbs should be the size of your fist (about 40 to 50 grams per meal or 20 to 25 grams per snack).

- **Veggies:** Eat as many naked ones as you like (check out the list of Real-Food Hunger Busters on page 185), but if they're cooked in something that adds fat, like butter or olive oil, the rule changes. In that case, a normal portion is $^1/_4$ to $^1/_2$ cup.

- **Fat:** A portion of fat is equivalent to the size of a golf ball about 15 grams per meal or 10 grams per snack. But if you eat fat from a real-food source, don't be worried if you consume more than the allotted amount. Also, don't stress if you consume more than the recommended daily amount of coconut oil (see below). The amount of calories it takes for the body to burn off the coconut oil is higher than the amount of calories in the coconut oil, which means that coconut oil boosts your metabolism.

- **Snacks:** Keep them small. For instance, if you're going to have nuts as a snack, stop at a handful, don't fill a bowl and pig out.

- **Fruit:** Fruit is an amazing source of fiber and vitamins, but remember that some fruits are pretty high in sugar and too much of one of these might kick off a sugar craving. Just be sure that every time you eat fruit, you eat it with protein in a PC combo or with a fat in an FC combo. *Tip: Dried fruit is especially high in sugar, so follow the same rule as when eating any snack: Keep it to a handful and combine it with a protein or fat.*

- *Very high in sugar:* tangerines, cherries, grapes, pomegranates, mangos, figs, bananas, dried fruit
- *Fairly high in sugar:* plums, oranges, kiwifruit, pears, pineapple
- *Low to moderate sugar:* strawberries, papaya, watermelon, peaches, nectarines, blueberries, cantaloupe, honeydew, apples, guavas, apricots, grapefruit
- *Lowest in sugar:* raspberries, cranberries, lemon, lime, rhubarb

- **Still hungry?** Drink a cup of warm tea (decaf or regular). If you continue to feel hunger pangs, eat a serving of nonstarchy food. (See Real-Food Hunger Busters on page 185.)

Other Foods to Try

In addition to the fiber-filled and omega-3-rich foods that will form the basis of your PC and FC combo meals, there are a few other foods I suggest you add to your diet.

- **Consume 2 tablespoons of virgin cold-pressed coconut oil** to kickstart your metabolism. I recommend 1 tablespoon of virgin coconut oil in tea, warm water, or black coffee in the morning to boost metabolic rate, immunity, and nutrient absorption, improve skin, liver function, and kidney function, reduce harmful yeast, and lessen hunger. Take 1 tablespoon of virgin coconut oil in $^1/_4$ cup warm water before bed for all the benefits previously listed and to help you sleep better. It really works. I do it every night! (See How Coconut Oil Aids in Weight Loss on page 169.)

- **Consume one serving of a fermented food per day** such as coconut water kefir (page 204), dairy kefir, kombucha tea, homemade sauerkraut (page 226), kimchi (made without MSG), Siggi's Probiotic drinkable fat-free yogurt, or Healing Movement Raw Cultured Vegetables. (See What's So Great about

Fermentation? on page 170 for the benefits of fermentation for weight loss.)

- **Add fat-melting foods to your menu,** like seaweed, seaweed flakes, vinegar, coconut oil, omega-3 rich foods, vitamin C rich foods, cinnamon, high fiber foods, cayenne pepper, garlic, and ginger. (See Fat-Burning Foods to Add to your Real-Food Diet on page 171 for more information.)

- **Drink 8 to 10 glasses of water per day** to help digest fibrous foods and avoid hunger pangs.

How Many Calories Should I Be Eating?

As I've said, when you're eating mostly real food, you shouldn't need to count calories to reach your weight loss goals. In any case, the amount of calories you need varies depending on your height, build, activity level, and amount of weight you want to lose. However, as a general rule of thumb, to lose weight most adult women should be eating about 1,500 calories per day; most men, about 2,000 calories per day.

My Best Real-Food Weight Loss Tips for Setting Yourself Up for Success

One of the things I try to hammer home to my clients is that to lose weight you have to set yourself up for success. It's you against the enticing, fattening, convenient food-filled world out there, and the only way to avoid falling into old bad habits is to be prepared. Here are a few tips that will help you set yourself up for success.

A MOVEABLE FEAST

Invest in some great food storage containers. On this diet plan you're going to have to pack and go quite often, especially when it comes to lunch and snacks. Having a great storage system helps keep you organized and enables you to take your real food on the go. Here are two of my favorites when it comes to food storage.

- Frigoverre Fun Food Storage (available at Target or The Container Store).

- French Bull storage containers (available at www.frenchbull.com). They are a bit of a splurge, but they'll last forever.

An adult lunch kit is also a must! My faves:

- Plastica Bento Box (available at www.plasticashop.com).

- Samfe Insulated Neoprene Lunch Tote with Separate Bottle and Food Sections (available on Amazon.com).

WEEKENDS ARE MADE FOR PRECOOKING AND PREPPING

Cook and prep foods on the weekends. It's easier then to shop and spend time preparing foods that you can easily grab to go during the week. Here are some of my favorite precooking tips:

- Bake about six sweet potatoes on the weekend, and store them in the fridge. This will give you quick and easy access to a fantastic real-food carbohydrate source to add to lunch or dinner or even have with breakfast. I often have a sweet potato on the side of my scrambled eggs when I don't have toast. I also hard-cook a dozen cage free omega-3 eggs so I have a simple grab-and-go protein to pair with a carbohydrate if I need it. Plus, I often find myself eating a hard-cooked egg with a grapefruit or banana as an afternoon snack.

- Roast a whole chicken or turkey to use in tacos, soups, sandwiches, and wraps during the week. These days, you can even find inexpensive free range roasted chickens or half chickens at many natural food supermarkets.

- Stock up on frozen vegetables and fruits for side dishes or smoothies. Although it's great to purchase fresh fruits and vegetables from your local farmers' market, frozen fruits and vegetables are a fantastic alternative because they're usually frozen within hours of being harvested.

- Precook oatmeal and put it in the fridge in single-serving containers. While it's cooking, add cinnamon, nutmeg, and a tiny bit of clove or allspice. In the morning I microwave it and add some coconut or soy milk and it's ready to go.

- Other great foods to prepare in advance include tuna fish salad (a great source of omega-3s!), egg salad, and chopped veggies for salads.

- Use prewashed baby spinach for many of your salads. It's so, *so* much easier and faster than washing lettuce. Leave the fancy lettuces for when you have more time.

SPLURGE ON A MIND-BLOWING VINEGAR

Buy a bottle of *good* delicious vinegar. If the vinegar is fantastic, it's all you'll need on a veggie salad. Splurge here and I promise you'll make up for it in pounds lost from skipping fatty salad dressing. An outstanding fig balsamic or tasty champagne vinegar beats a fat-laden salad dressing any day. I've found that it's fun to shop for good vinegar at Williams-Sonoma because you can often taste it before you buy it. In addition, the Web site www.napavalleyproducts.com sells some of my all-time favorite vinegars, including an amazing Zinfandel Vinegar and Strawberry Balsamic Vinegar.

How Coconut Oil Aids in Weight Loss

For decades many of us were told that coconut oil was a harmful saturated fat. However, as has been the case for so much of the nutrition advice doled out in the 20th century, that information is flat out wrong. The truth is that coconut oil is one of the healthiest fats around. The traditional cultures that consume coconuts and coconut oil have some of the lowest rates of heart disease in the world, not to mention they're some of the slimmest people on the globe.

In 1998, obesity researchers at McGill University found that medium chain fatty acids (MCFAs), the type found in coconuts, actually use up energy when they are metabolized. The calories the body uses to oxidize the fatty acids in coconut oil is greater than the calories they provide. So it's possible to burn more calories digesting coconut oil than you get from eating it. In addition, coconut oil has a so-called "thermogenic effect," which means it raises your body temperature, thus boosting your metabolism and energy level. This is another property behind the weight loss effect of coconut oil.

Another great benefit of coconut oil is that it's a highly stable oil, so you can keep it unrefrigerated in your pantry for years and it will not go rancid. It remains stable even at very high temperatures, making it the ideal cooking oil. I recommend that you use coconut oil any time a recipe calls for cooking oil or shortening.

One final fascinating fact about coconut oil: The primary fatty acid in coconut oil, lauric acid, which is highly antiviral, antibacterial, and antifungal, is also found in human breast milk—which, let's face it, is the perfect food!

What's So Great about Fermentation?

Fermentation increases the flavor, medicinal value, and nutrition of foods. Pickling, brewing, and culturing are other terms used to describe this process by which friendly enzymes, fungi, and bacteria predigest a food. Because overprocessing can kill the healthy bacteria in fermented foods, you must be sure to buy quality "living" fermented foods.

These living fermented foods boost the immune system by increasing antibodies that fight infectious disease. The flora in living fermented foods form a shield that covers the small intestine's inner lining and helps inhibit pathogenic organisms, including E. coli, salmonella, and an unhealthy overgrowth of yeast. Some fermented foods even create antioxidants that fight free radicals, a precursor to cancer. In addition, fermentation transforms hard-to-digest lactose from milk to the more easily digested lactic acid. Yogurt is an example of this process.

Finally, fermentation can neutralize the antinutrients found in many foods, including the phytic acid found in all grains and the trypsin-inhibitors in soy. (An antinutrient is a substance that binds to vitamins, minerals, and enzymes to make them unavailable to the body.) And fermentation generates new nutrients, including omega-3 fatty acids (for example, when soy is fermented to make miso) and digestive aids like the enzyme diastase.

So do fermented foods speed up weight loss? Not necessarily, but they will *support* weight loss. Here's why: For one thing, fermented foods do tend to be nutritionally dense and filling, and some are low calorie. In addition, the probiotic nature of some fermented foods aids in the digestion of food and assimilation of nutrients.

The living cultured foods commercially available include some brands of kefir, yogurt, miso, tofu, sauerkraut, and kimchi (Korean pickled vegetables). As I mentioned on the previous page, some fermented foods are available at Whole Food's Market, such as Siggi's Probiotic drinkable fat-free yogurt and Healing Movement Raw Cultured Vegetables. Check out my Homemade Sauerkraut recipe on page 226.

Fat-Burning Foods to Add to Your Real-Food Diet

Artichoke: *Artichokes contain inulin, which is a type of carbohydrate that has been shown to decrease the hunger hormone ghrelin.*

Cayenne pepper: *Cayenne pepper heats up the body and therefore is thought to increase metabolism. Chili pepper has a similar effect.*

Cinnamon: *According to the USDA, consuming as little as a ¼ teaspoon of cinnamon with food helps the body metabolize sugar 20 times faster and lowers blood sugar levels. This means faster weight loss!*

Ginger: *Ginger has been found to increase feelings of satiety.*

Seaweed: *The property in seaweed that helps us lose weight is alginate, which lines the walls of the digestive system and prevents dietary fat from passing through.*

Tea: *The caffeine in tea stimulates thermogenesis, the biochemical process by which fat in the body is burned to produce energy. Plus, tea has a fabulous antioxidant called EGCG (Epigallocatechin gallate) that provides fat burning activity.*

Vinegar: *Vinegar helps lower blood glucose levels.*

The Real-Food Diet Weight Loss Meal Plan

Now that you understand how replacing fake factory foods with real food will lead to weight loss and you've learned how to find great real food, it's time to put your real-food weight loss diet into action. For maximum weight loss, remember to follow the real-food weight loss rules outlined on page 159.

The 2-week sample meal plan below is an example of how to put all of this together. All the meals are high in fiber and omega-3s, with a minimum of refined sugar, refined carbs, salt, and additives. They are mostly PCF combos, with the snacks mostly PC or FC combos, in reasonable portions. As you'll see, the meal plans do allow you to eat out, but also encourage you to get in the kitchen and use recipes that are low in calories yet high in flavor. You'll find the complete recipes in Chapter 12. Some of the recipes make more than one serving, but for the meals below, you'll just eat one serving and save the leftovers for later meals, so you don't have to cook for every meal.

In order to make sure you're getting real food every 4 hours or so, the meal plans call for three meals plus a snack. Feel free to jump around with the meal plans on the next few pages and have breakfast for dinner, or lunch for breakfast, whatever works for you. You can also add snacks and hunger busters (page 185) if you need to in order to help with the timing of your meals. Repeat days over and over if you don't feel like cooking up all of these recipes. And I encourage you to experiment and make substitutions in the recipes if you'd like. As long as you have a nice variety of real foods, feel free to eat whatever works for you. Just make sure whatever you eat is real food, that you're getting all of the fiber and omega-3s you need and none of the refined carbs you don't, and follow these guidelines:

- Avoid packaged food with artificial ingredients and preservatives as much as humanly possible.
- Drink 8 to 10 glasses of water per day to help digest fibrous foods and avoid hunger pangs.
- Have one tablespoon of virgin coconut oil in the morning, one in the evening. Mix it in a $1/4$ cup of warm water, tea, or black coffee.
- Eat or drink one $1/2$ cup serving of a fermented food per day, at a time of day that is convenient for you. Note: It does not have to be with a meal. You can eat your fermented food whenever you want, because it does not affect blood sugar levels negatively.
- Add fat-melting foods as appropriate.

DAY ONE

Breakfast: 1 Lemony Blueberry Muffin (page 195) with one 7-ounce container Siggi's Icelandic Style Skyr Strained Non-Fat Yogurt, the traditional yogurt of Iceland. It's full of protein and contains no fat.

Lunch (dining out): grilled chicken sandwich on a whole wheat bun (no cheese), lettuce, tomato, onion, and a side of fruit

Snack: 1 Lemony Blueberry Muffin (page 195) with one 7-ounce container of of Siggi's Skyr

Dinner: Cilantro-Lime Shrimp with Spicy Rice Noodles (page 244) Note: Prepare 10 extra shrimp for lunch tomorrow.

DAY TWO

Breakfast: Açai Superfood Smoothie (page 207)

Lunch: Greek Isles Salad (page 224) with shrimp from day 1 dinner

Snack: 1 Purple Passion Quesadilla (page 260) with Fire Roasted Salsa Verde (page 258). Save leftovers for a snack on day 4.

Dinner: Farmers' Market "Tortilla" Soup (page 213). Note: Save leftovers for lunch tomorrow.

DAY THREE

Breakfast: Canadian Sunrise Sandwich (page 199)

Lunch: Farmers' Market "Tortilla" Soup from day 2 dinner

Snack: Ole Guacamole (page 261) and Skinny Chips (page 259). Save leftover chips for Day 6 snack.

Dinner: Grilled Margarita Pizza (page 242) with Arugula and Beet Salad (page 216)

DAY FOUR

Breakfast: Fizzie Fruit Smoothie (page 211)

Lunch (dining out): Chipotle Burrito Bowl with chicken or steak, black beans, salsa, corn, and guac (split it with a friend—the whole bowl is over 700 calories, and you don't need that)

Snack: 1 Purple Passion Quesadilla (page 260) with Fire Roasted Salsa Verde (page 258) from day 2 snack

Dinner: Mongolian Beef (page 235). Save leftovers for lunch tomorrow.

DAY FIVE

Breakfast: Two European Yogurts (available at Trader Joe's or Whole Foods)

Lunch: Mongolian Beef (page 235) from day 4 dinner

Snack: Spiced Up Egg Salad (page 225) with 2 slices of Ezekiel bread

Dinner: Easy Lobster Pasta (page 243). Save leftovers for lunch tomorrow.

DAY SIX

Breakfast: 1 slice Bangin' Banana Bread (page 201) with 2 hard-cooked organic cage free omega-3 eggs

Lunch: Easy Lobster Pasta (page 243) from day 5 dinner

Snack: Fire Roasted Salsa Verde (page 258) with Skinny Chips (page 259) from day 2 and day 3 snacks.

Dinner: Citrus-Soaked Pork Tacos (page 238)

DAY SEVEN

Breakfast: South of the Border Scramble (page 196) with beef bacon and Fire Roasted Salsa Verde (page 258) and 4 dried or fresh figs

Lunch: Make a salad using leftover pork from day 6 dinner. Add iceberg lettuce, black olives, tomato, green onion, and top with Fire Roasted Salsa Verde (page 258).

Snack: 2 medium slices of melon wrapped with 2 slices of prosciutto (Applegate Farms is the best, unless you buy imported)

Dinner: Farmers' Market Veggie Pasta (page 246), Arugula and Beet Salad (page 216)

DAY ONE

Breakfast: Jeweled Steel-Cut Oats (page 203)

Lunch: Italian Lentil Soup (page 214) with Tuscan Kale Toss (page 220) and Homemade Croutons (page 221). Save leftover soup for snack tomorrow.

Snack: Santorini Lemon-Feta Dip (page 256) with Whole Wheat Pita Chips (page 257)

Dinner: Ruby Yakitori Kababs (page 231), Cucumber Salad with Yuzu and Sesame (page 218) and Asian Quinoa Salad (page 222)

DAY TWO

Breakfast: Razzy Peach Parfait (page 206)

Lunch: 1 cup Butternut Sage Soup (page 212)

Snack: 1 cup Italian Lentil Soup from day 1 lunch

Dinner: Herb Crusted Rack of Lamb with Açai Sauce (page 240) with fingerling roasted garlic potatoes (page 181) and steamed broccoli

DAY THREE

Breakfast: Coconut "Faux"gurt (page 205) with 1 cup fresh raspberries

Lunch: Autumn Harvest Salad (page 223)

Snack: Caprese salad: 1 ounce fresh mozzarella, fresh basil, sliced tomato, extra-virgin olive oil, and sea salt

Dinner: Roasted Vegetable Lasagna (page 247) and russet potatoes. Save leftovers for lunch tomorrow.

DAY FOUR

Breakfast: Petite Asparagus Frittatas (page 197) with a medium peach. Save leftovers for snack tomorrow.

Lunch: Roasted Vegetable Lasagna from day 3 dinner

Snack: Avocado-Tomato Salad (page 217) with a tangerine

Dinner: Minted Greek Chicken (page 230). Save some chicken for lunch tomorrow.

DAY FIVE

Breakfast: Fresh Baked Granola (page 202)

Lunch: Arugula and Beet Salad (page 216) with pomegranate seeds and leftover Minted Greek Chicken from day 4 dinner

Snack: 1 Petite Asparagus Frittata from day 4 with ½ cup pomegranate seeds

Dinner: Chef Cece's Bouillabaisse (page 234) with 1 small toasted sourdough baguette from your local bakery. Save leftovers for snack tomorrow.

DAY SIX

Breakfast: Rustic German Apple Pancake (page 200)

Lunch: Heirloom Mac 'n' Cheese Muffins (page 262) with Quick Tomato Soup (page 215). Save leftovers for snack tomorrow.

Snack: 1 cup leftover Chef Cece's Bouillabaisse from day 5 with 1 small slice sourdough bread from your local bakery

Dinner: Grilled Halibut with Tomato Coulis (page 232) with spinach salad with balsamic vinaigrette. To make vinaigrette, use one part vinegar to two parts extra-virgin olive oil, whisk rapidly and, drizzle over fresh spinach leaves. Save leftovers for lunch tomorrow.

DAY SEVEN

Breakfast: Cremini-Mozza Quiche (page 198)

Lunch: Grilled Halibut with Tomato Coulis from day 6 dinner with ½ cup cooked quinoa or brown rice

Snack: Heirloom Mac 'n' Cheese Muffins (page 262) with Quick Tomato Soup (page 215) from day 6 lunch

Dinner: Smoky Beef Stew (page 236)

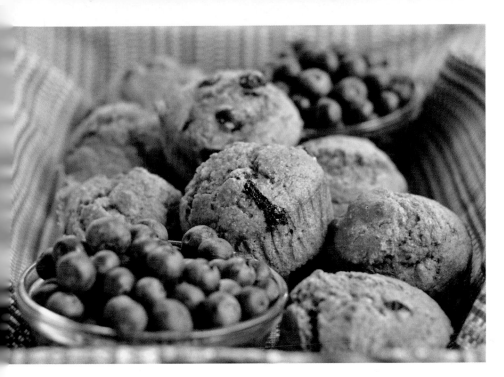

Lemony Blueberry Muffins (page 195)

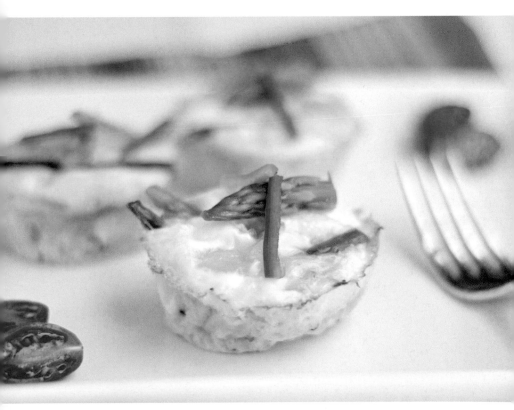

Petite Asparagus Frittatas (page 197)

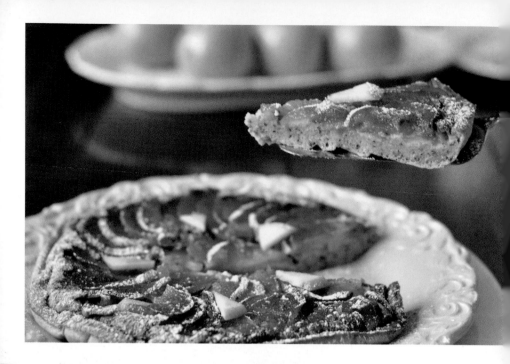

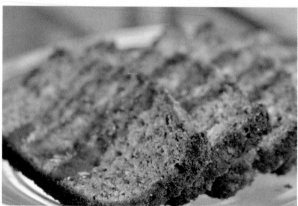

Rustic German Apple Pancake (page 200)

Bangin' Banana Bread (page 201)

Jeweled Steel-Cut Oats (page 203)

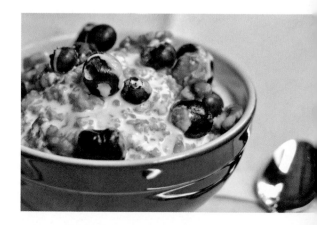

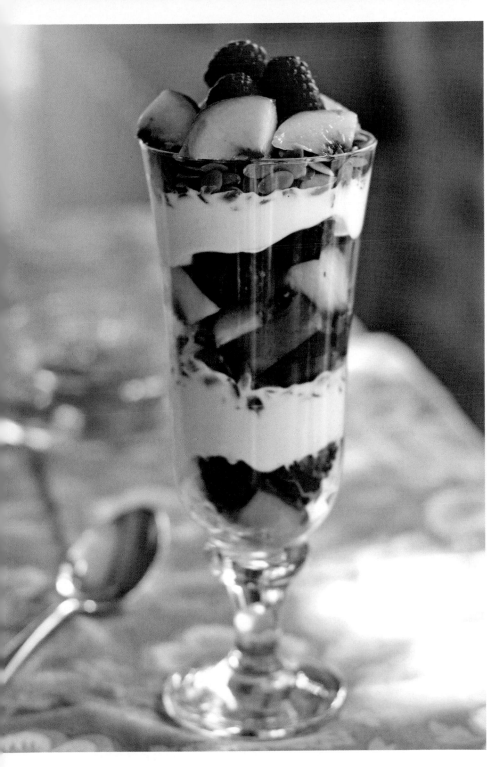

Razzy Peach Parfait (page 206)

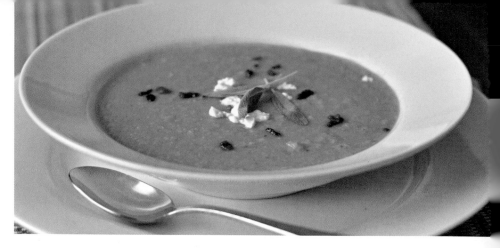

Butternut Sage Soup (page 212)

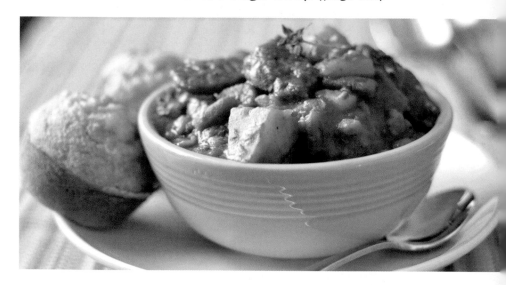

Smoky Beef Stew (page 236) **and**
Chipotle Cheddar Cornbread (page 237)

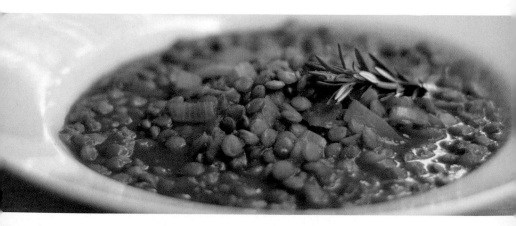

Italian Lentil Soup (page 214)

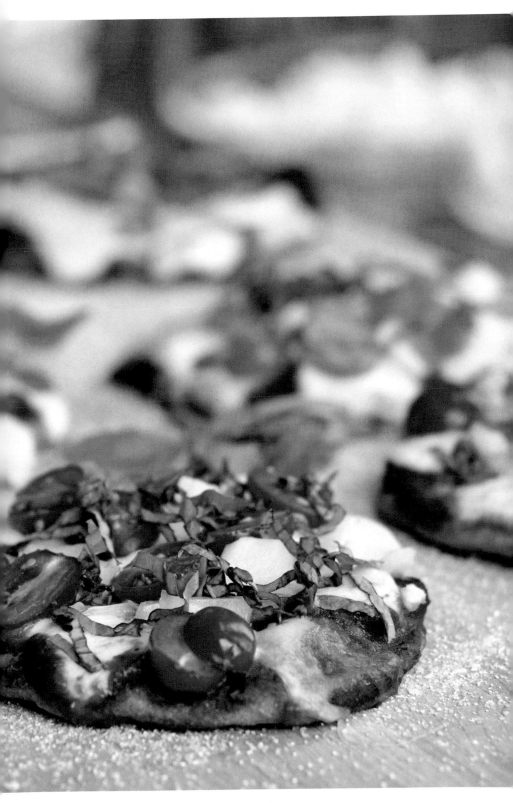

Grilled Margarita Pizzas (page 242)

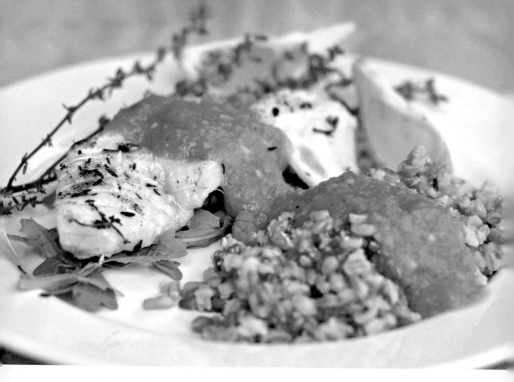

Grilled Halibut with Tomato Coulis (page 232)

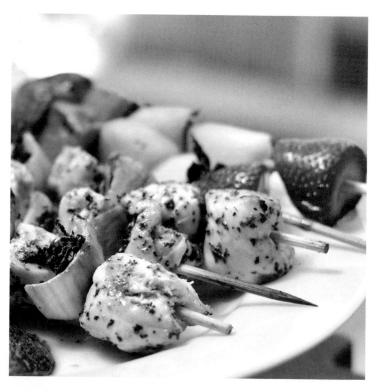

Minted Greek Chicken (page 230)

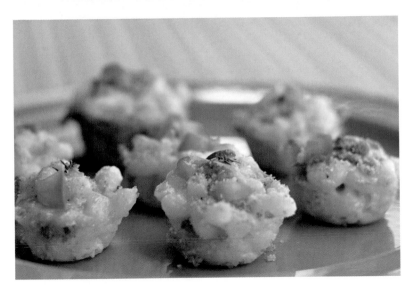

Heirloom Mac 'n' Cheese Muffins (page 262)

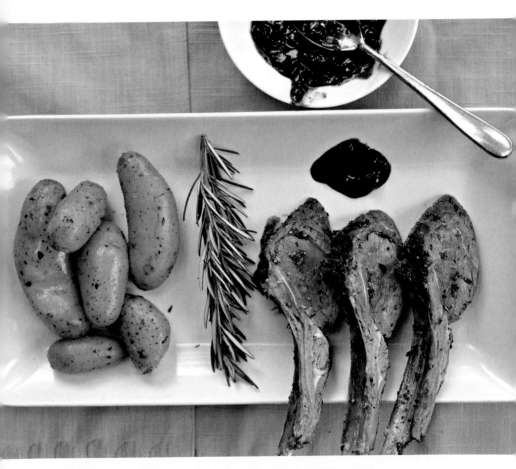

Herb-Crusted Rack of Lamb with Açaí Sauce (page 240)

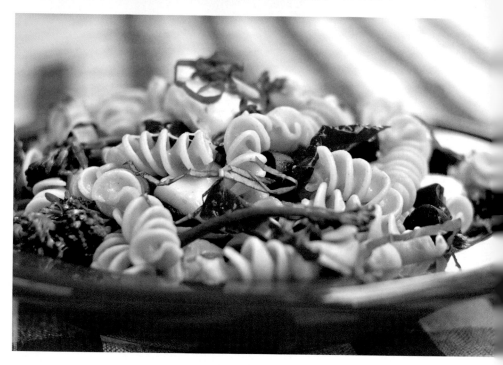

Farmers' Market Veggie Pasta (page 246)

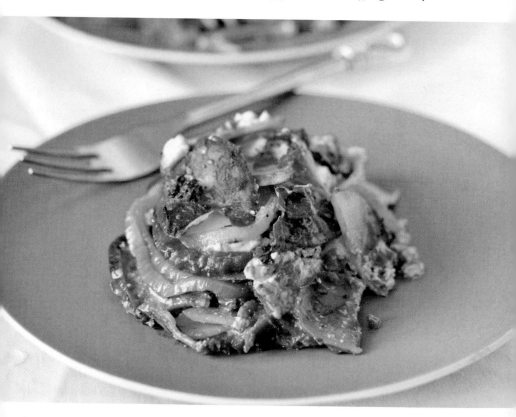

Roasted Vegetable Lasagna (page 247)

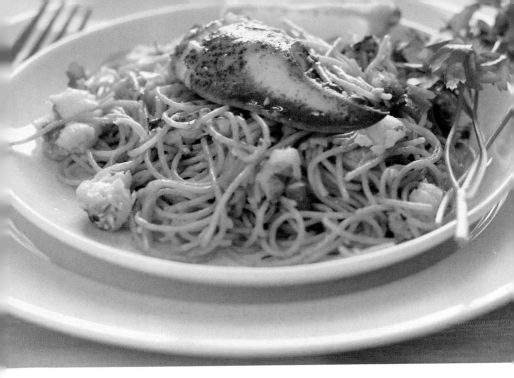

Easy Lobster Pasta (page 243)

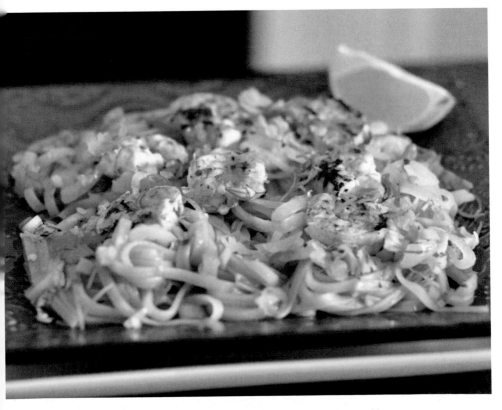

Cilantro-Lime Shrimp with Spicy Rice Noodles (page 244)

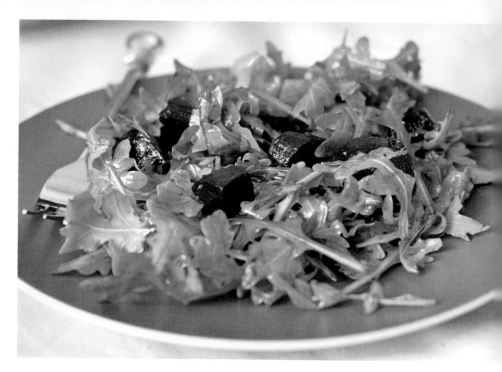

Arugula and Beet Salad (page 216)

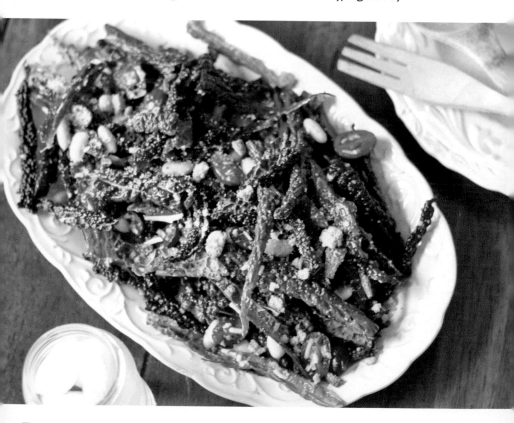

Tuscan Kale Toss (page 220) **and Homemade Croutons** (page 221)

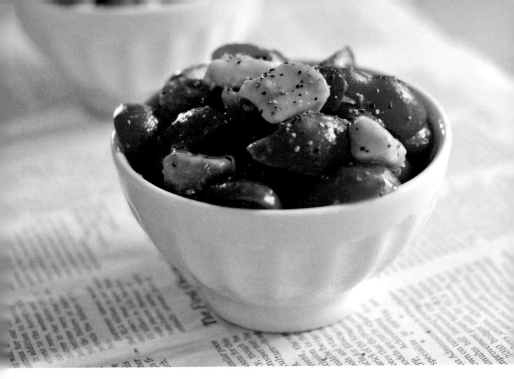

Avocado-Tomato Salad (page 217)

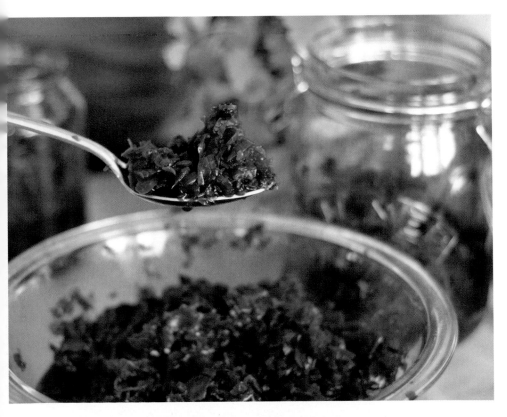

Homemade Sauerkraut (page 226)

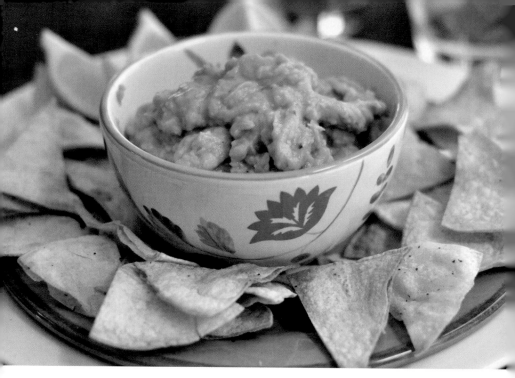

Olé Guacamole (page 261) **and Skinny Chips** (page 259)

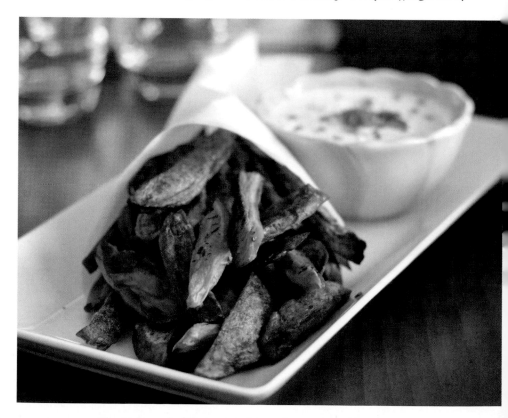

Purple and Sweet Potato Fries (page 264)

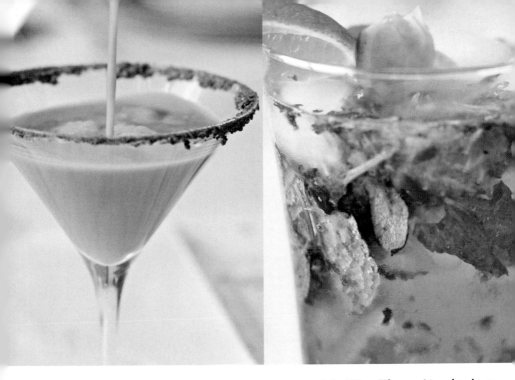

Espresso Martini (page 265)

Mojito Flaquito (a.k.a. Skinny Mojito) (page 266)

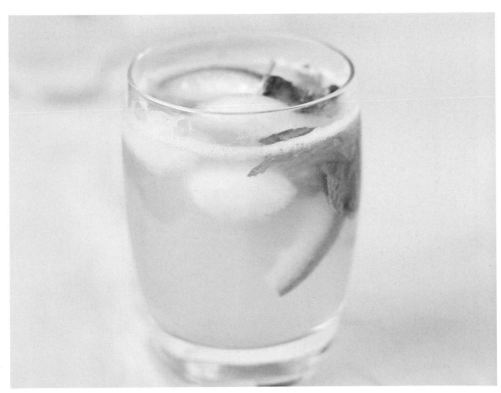

Pomelo Martini (page 267)

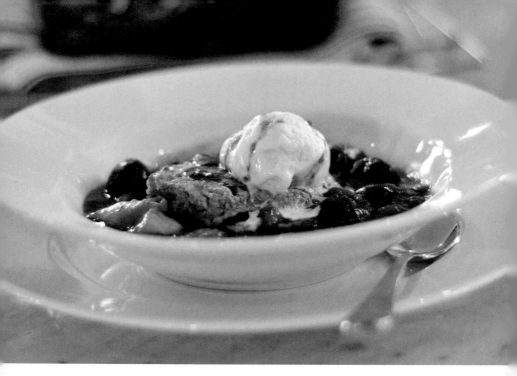

White Peach and Bing Cherry Cobbler (page 252)

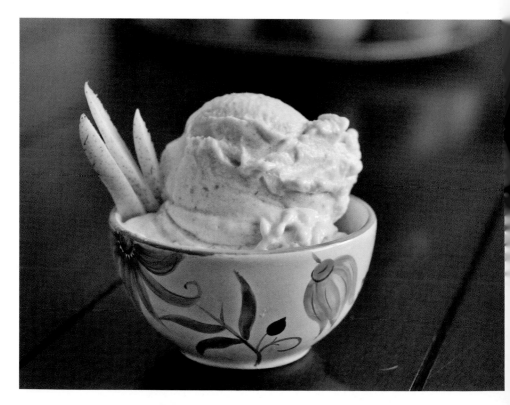

Tipsy Pear Sorbet (page 255)

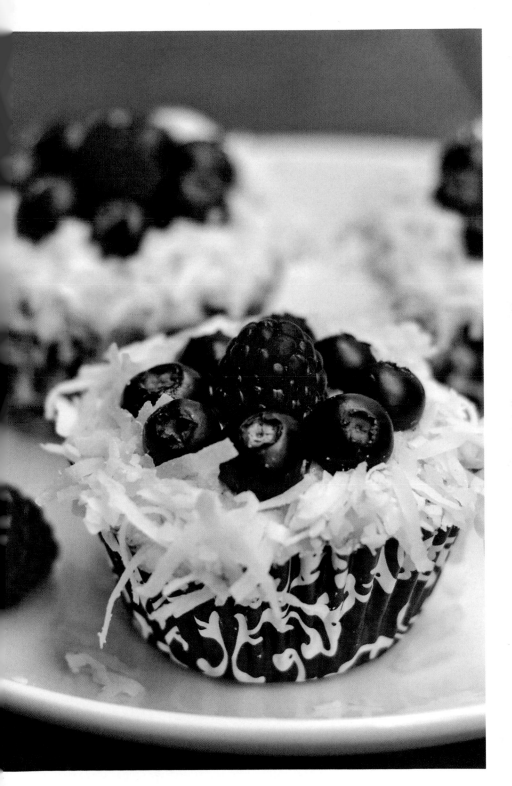

Cocoberry Cupcakes (page 250)

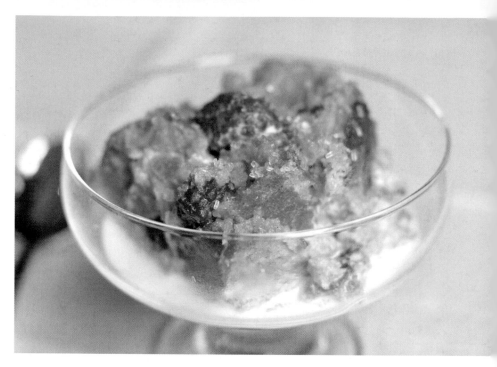

Lemonata Raspberry Bread Pudding (page 248)

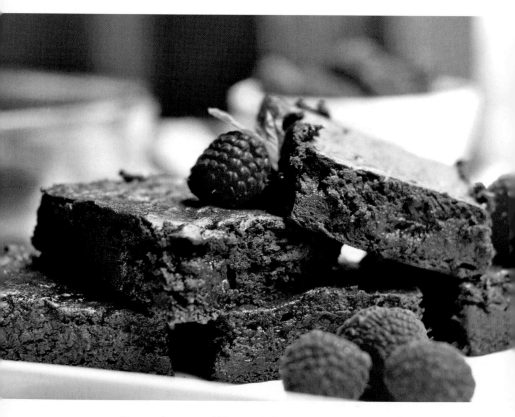

Raspberry-Kissed Brownies (page 249)

Real-Food Fat Blaster Plan

Now for a little *lagniappe*, New Orleans (one of my favorite real-food cities!) lingo for "a little something extra." I've developed a second real-food weight loss plan for folks who need to lose weight on the fast track. I was inspired to develop this plan after working with several clients who wanted to lose weight fast for a particular event or goal, like bikini season or their big day walking down the aisle.

I call it the Real-Food Fat Blaster plan. For the most part, it's a factory food detox. So you can use it for the first week of your official real-food weight loss diet (and then go on to the 2-week meal plan on pages 173 to 176). There are zero factory foods in this plan, and the food preparation is simple and very straightforward. There are no elaborate recipes in this plan. It is designed to help you lose weight as quickly as possible with simple, quick, and easy food preparation. It's a great transition to your real-food weight loss lifestyle.

If you get hungry between lunch and dinner, choose a snack from the list at the end of the menu. The plan is designed to get you into a real-food mode. Most of these meals can be made in less than 10 minutes. Below are my guidelines for the plan.

- Eat one serving of a fermented food you like or drink ½ cup of a fermented beverage per day. If you prefer to consume more, be mindful of the calories and try not to exceed 80 calories of fermented foods per day.
  - Homemade Sauerkraut (page 226)
  - Kombucha
  - Kimchi
  - Dairy kefir
  - Coconut Water Kefir (page 204)
  - Siggi's Probiotic drinkable fat-free yogurt (all real ingredients!) (available at Whole Foods)
  - Healing Movement Raw Cultured Vegetables
- Consume at least one serving of food that contains omega-3s,

such as one 3-ounce serving of a fatty fish like salmon, per day, or take an omega-3 supplement. Do not buy a supplement that contains omega-3, omega-6, and omega-9; that would be a waste of money because Americans get more than enough of the latter two.

- Drink Christine's Detox Tea (page 269) or any green tea throughout the day or consume a minimum of 2 cups of tea per day.

- Consume 2 tablespoons of virgin cold-pressed coconut oil per day.

WEEK ONE

DAY ONE

Breakfast options: PB&J toast with berries and a hard-cooked egg (my personal weekday breakfast)

> 2 slices of Ezekiel Bread (or gluten free bread)
>
> 1 tablespoon organic all-natural peanut butter
>
> 1 tablespoon homemade or farmers' market preserves (I love Bouncing Berry Farms organic fruit delight— all-natural, nothing fake, sweetened with agave)
>
> 1 hard-cooked egg, free range (look for the eggs that say "omega-3" on the package)
>
> ½ cup in-season organic berries
>
> 1 tablespoon organic expeller-pressed coconut oil in 1 cup of green tea or coffee (if you prefer it sweet, sweeten only with stevia)

Lunch: Grilled salmon with a Mediterranean salad

> **Salmon:** 1 piece grilled salmon (purchase prepared from Whole Foods or other local market)

To make grilled salmon: Brush salmon lightly with extra-virgin olive oil, season with sea salt, pepper, and your favorite herbs and spices. Grill over medium-high heat for 4 minutes on each side. If you have a fish griller, this will be very quick and easy. If you don't have a grill, place salmon on a baking sheet covered with foil and bake at 400°F for 10 to

12 minutes, turning once halfway through, or until desired doneness.

Salad: 1 cup spinach leaves, ¼ cup diced red bell pepper, 1 tablespoon low-fat feta, ⅓ cup organic chickpeas, ⅓ cup cannellini beans, 1 tablespoon balsamic vinaigrette

Dinner: Grilled steak topped with baby bellas and sweet onions, with baked potato and asparagus

4 ounces grilled grass fed steak topped with ¼ cup sautéed sweet onions and 4 baby bella mushrooms

To make grilled steak: Once steak is room temperature, coat with extra-virgin olive oil, sea salt, pepper, and your favorite herbs and spices. For a one-inch-thick steak served medium: grill over medium-high heat for 6 minutes on one side and 4 minutes on the other side. Done when internal temperature registers 140°F to 150°F.

To make potato: Heat oven to 350°F. Wash, and poke 8 to 12 holes deep into the potato. Lightly coat with extra-virgin olive oil, sea salt, and pepper. Place in the middle of the oven and bake for 1 hour, until the outer layer of the potato is slightly crispy but the flesh feels soft. Garnish with a teaspoon of sour cream and a sprinkle of sliced chives.

To make asparagus spears: Lightly coat asparagus spears with extra-virgin olive oil, sea salt, and pepper. Place in oven with potato during the last 25 minutes of baking time.

Evening: 1 tablespoon organic expeller-pressed coconut oil in decaf tea or warm water

DAY TWO

Breakfast: Banana Coconut Yogurt Smoothie

1 cup light coconut milk, chilled

2 tablespoons flaxseed meal (I love Barlean's)

1 large banana

1 tablespoon coconut oil

One 7-ounce container of low-fat or fat-free Greek yogurt

Mix in blender for about 1–2 minutes or until desired consistency.

Lunch: Chicken sandwich and baby spinach salad

Sweet caramelized onion chicken patty (from Costco or Sam's Club; read ingredient label—must be 100 percent real food)

Served on an Ezekiel bun topped with lettuce, tomato, red onion, and Dijon mustard.

1 large apple, sliced and sprinkled with cinnamon.

Baby spinach (or watercress or arugula) salad with balsamic vinegar and extra-virgin olive oil.

Dinner: Roasted turkey, lima beans, and mixed berries

Palm-size slice of oven roasted turkey breast. Buy premade at Whole Foods or other local market or make it at home

1 cup lima beans, frozen, heated in saucepan with herbes de Provence

1 cup mixed berries with fresh mint

1 tablespoon organic expeller-pressed coconut oil in decaf tea or warm water

DAY THREE

Breakfast: Breakfast burrito

1 whole wheat Ezekiel tortilla stuffed with 2 free range scrambled eggs; 2 cherry tomatoes, diced; handful of sunflower sprouts (or any sprout you like); 1/3 avocado

1 tablespoon organic expeller-pressed coconut oil in 1 cup of green tea (if you prefer it sweet, sweeten only with stevia)

Lunch: Quick tuna sandwich

1 small can chunky light tuna, 1 tablespoon each of preservative-free real mayonnaise, diced dill pickle, diced celery

2 slices Ezekiel bread

1 cup organic grapes

Dinner: Grilled lamb chops, fingerling potatoes, arugula salad

To grill lamb chops: Heat outdoor grill to medium-high heat. Lightly coat lamb chops with olive oil, rub with minced garlic, fresh minced rosemary, and fresh minced oregano. Once chops are room temperature, place them on the grill for 3 to 4 minutes per side. If you do not have an outdoor grill, preheat your oven to 400ºF. Sear chops in a heatproof frying pan with a teaspoon of olive oil for 1 minute on each side. Move frying pan to oven and roast for 10 minutes.

To make potatoes: Toss 5 fingerling potatoes with olive oil, garlic, and rosemary. Roast in oven at 500ºF for 25 minutes.

1 cup arugula with 1 tablespoon balsamic vinaigrette

1 tablespoon organic expeller-pressed coconut oil in decaf tea or warm water

DAY FOUR

Breakfast: Greek yogurt parfait

One 7-ounce container of low-fat Greek yogurt mixed with 1 cup organic berries (fresh or frozen), and a small handful of raw nuts

1 tablespoon organic expeller-pressed coconut oil in 1 cup of green tea (if you prefer it sweet, sweeten only with stevia)

Lunch: Leftover lamb chops and arugula salad

2 leftover grilled lamb chops

1 cup arugula with 1 tablespoon balsamic vinaigrette

1 medium bowl of cubed melon (watermelon, honeydew, or cantaloupe)

Dinner: Top sirloin burger with baby spinach salad

To make burgers: In a medium mixing bowl, combine 1 pound grass fed ground sirloin beef with 1 tablespoon Annie's Naturals Worcestershire sauce, sea salt, and pepper. Sauté a diced medium onion in 1 teaspoon extra-virgin olive oil and add to the beef mixture. Form four patties. Toast Ezekiel buns in frying pan. Cook patties in frying pan with

1 teaspoon of extra-virgin olive oil. Serve with organic ketchup, mustard, lettuce, and tomato.

To make salad: Toss organic baby spinach with 1 diced bell pepper, cherry tomatoes, and shredded carrots and drizzle with vinegar and extra-virgin olive oil.

1 tablespoon organic expeller-pressed coconut oil in decaf tea or warm water

DAY FIVE

Breakfast: Yogurt Espresso Shake

1 cup light coconut milk, chilled

1 shot espresso (if you don't have an espresso maker, use coffee)

1 tablespoon coconut oil

One 7-ounce container low-fat Greek yogurt

Lunch:

2 leftover sirloin burgers

1 cup baby spinach with 1 tablespoon balsamic vinaigrette

1 medium baked sweet potato that you cooked in advance

Dinner:

EVOL frozen burrito (available at most Whole Foods)

Medium orange

1 tablespoon organic expeller-pressed coconut oil in decaf tea or warm water

DAY SIX

Breakfast:

2 scrambled free range eggs, fresh salsa, $\frac{1}{3}$ cup black beans, 1 Ezekiel tortilla

1 tablespoon organic expeller-pressed coconut oil in 1 cup of green tea (if you prefer it sweet, sweeten only with stevia)

Lunch: Asian salad

To make salad: Combine grilled chicken breast or roasted poultry leftover from earlier in the week, shredded farmers' market cabbage, 1 tablespoon sliced almonds, tangerine sections, snap peas, red onion, ½ cup cooked quinoa, olive oil, and rice vinegar.

Dinner: Salmon with sweet potato and steamed broccolini

To make salmon: Lightly coat salmon with extra-virgin olive oil and rub with garlic, rosemary, sea salt, and pepper. Roast in oven at 450°F for 5 minutes on each side.

Serve with 1 cup steamed broccolini (or broccoli) and a baked sweet potato that you made over the weekend.

1 tablespoon organic expeller-pressed coconut oil in decaf tea or warm water

DAY SEVEN

Breakfast: Pomegranate Peach Smoothie

1 cup light coconut milk, chilled

½ cup pomegranate seeds

1 medium peach, diced

1 tablespoon coconut oil

One 7-ounce container low-fat Greek yogurt

Lunch: Salmon wrap with apple

To make wrap: Wrap salmon left over from day 6 in an Ezekiel whole wheat tortilla with sprouts, arugula, carrot shreds, red onion, vinegar, and olive oil

1 medium apple

Dinner: Pasture raised organic pork tenderloin stir-fry with brown rice

To make stir-fry: In a medium bowl, combine 1 pound cubed pork tenderloin, 2 tablespoons soy sauce, 1 teaspoon ginger zest, 1 table-spoon minced garlic, 1 teaspoon Sriracha hot chili sauce and let sit for

10 minutes. *Prepare brown rice according to package directions. As rice is cooking, heat a large skillet or wok to medium-high heat with 1 tablespoon coconut oil. Stir-fry pork for 5 minutes. Add 1 cup snap peas, 1 tablespoon bamboo shoots, and 1 red bell pepper cut into thin julienne slices. Stir-fry for 2 more minutes. Serve with 1 cup brown rice.*

1 tablespoon organic expeller-pressed coconut oil in decaf tea or warm water

Fat Blaster Quick Snacks: (to be enjoyed between lunch and dinner)

16 cashews and a medium fruit

1 tablespoon natural peanut butter with 1 sliced apple

¼ cup hummus with 2 farmers' market carrots and 1 sliced bell pepper

1 ounce goat cheese spread on 2 small roasted beets

1 hard-cooked egg with a medium banana

1 fruit-flavored kombucha tea, 1 ounce dark chocolate, ½ cup berries

1 large orange with 1 ounce reduced fat smoked Gouda cheese (available at Trader Joe's)

Mini PB&J: 1 slice of Ezekiel bread (or gluten free bread), natural peanut butter, homemade preserves (or Bouncing Berry Farm Fruit Delight)

Real-Food Hunger Busters

I usually call these "free foods" because the suggested servings are less than 50 calories. Also, each food is so low in sugar that it won't be detrimental to blood sugar levels. They are great to add to your meals or eat between meals if you are hungry, because they won't spoil your weight loss efforts. Limit yourself to 1 cup raw or ½ cup cooked plain. Feel free to add a yummy vinegar.

Alfalfa sprouts

Artichokes

Asparagus

Bamboo shoots

Beet greens

Bok choy

Broccoli

Brussels sprouts

Cabbage (all varieties)

Cauliflower

Celery

Coleslaw (no dressing)

Collards

Cucumber

Eggplant

Garden salad (no dressing)

Green beans

Kale

Kohlrabi

Leeks

Lettuce

Mushrooms (all varieties)

Mustard greens

Okra

Onion (all varieties)

Parsley (all varieties)

Peppers (all varieties)

Pumpkin (fresh or canned)

Radicchio

Radish

Relish (not sweet)

Rutabaga

Sauerkraut (homemade or store bought without additives or preservatives)

Scallions

Spinach

Swiss chard

Tomatoes

Tomato paste

Tomato sauce

Turnips

Turnip greens

Watercress

Zucchini

Check It!

Below is a handy checklist to help you keep track of whether you're getting all the "must-eat" components of the plan. For additional checklists, log on to my Web site at www.christineavanti.com.

REAL-FOOD WEIGHT LOSS DIET DAILY CHECKLIST

Check off the item in the first blank and specify what it was in the longer blank.

MONDAY

_____ Fiber: 30 grams per day (equal to approximately 3 servings of fruit or 5 servings of vegetables per day; see the list of "excellent," "very good," and "good" sources of fiber on pages 162–163)._____

_____ Omega-3: minimum of 1 serving per day (see the list of "excellent" and "very good" sources of omega-3 on pages 163–164). _____

_____ Fermented food: once a day _____

_____ Coconut oil: 2 tablespoons per day _____

TUESDAY

_____ Fiber: 30 grams per day _____

_____ Omega-3: minimum of 1 serving per day _____

_____ Fermented food: once a day _____

_____ Coconut oil: 2 tablespoons per day _____

WEDNESDAY

_____ Fiber: 30 grams per day _____

_____ Omega-3: minimum of 1 serving per day _____

_____ Fermented food: once a day _____

_____ Coconut oil: 2 tablespoons per day _____

THURSDAY

_____ Fiber: 30 grams per day _____

_____ Omega-3: minimum of 1 serving per day _____

_____ Fermented food: once a day _____

_____ Coconut oil: 2 tablespoons per day _____

FRIDAY

_____ Fiber: 30 grams per day _____

_____ Omega-3: minimum of 1 serving per day _____

_____ Fermented food: once a day _____

_____ Coconut oil: 2 tablespoons per day _____

SATURDAY

_____ Fiber: 30 grams per day _____

_____

_____ Omega-3: minimum of 1 serving per day _____

_____

_____ Fermented food: once a day _____

_____

_____ Coconut oil: 2 tablespoons per day _____

_____

SUNDAY

_____ Fiber: 30 grams per day _____

_____

_____ Omega-3: minimum of 1 serving per day _____

_____

_____ Fermented food: once a day _____

_____

_____ Coconut oil: 2 tablespoons per day _____

_____

PC, FC, OR PFC COMBO AT EACH MEAL OR SNACK

Indicate whether each meal was a PC, FC, or PFC combo. A snack is either a PC or FC combo.

MONDAY
Breakfast_____ Lunch_____ Dinner_____ Snack_____ Snack_____

TUESDAY
Breakfast_____ Lunch_____ Dinner_____ Snack_____ Snack_____

WEDNESDAY
Breakfast_____ Lunch_____ Dinner_____ Snack_____ Snack_____

THURSDAY
Breakfast_____ Lunch_____ Dinner_____ Snack_____ Snack_____

FRIDAY

Breakfast____ Lunch____ Dinner____ Snack____ Snack____

SATURDAY

Breakfast____ Lunch____ Dinner____ Snack____ Snack____

SUNDAY

Breakfast____ Lunch____ Dinner____ Snack____ Snack____

Sunshine Boatwright: A Real-Foodie Weight Loss Story

Sunshine Boatwright, a 38-year-old woman from Dallas, Georgia, lost 81 pounds in 10 months after switching from a factory food diet to a real-food diet. Starting below is a conversation I had with Sunshine about her real-food weight loss.

When you made the switch from a factory food diet to a real-food diet were there any specific foods you had a hard time giving up? If so, what were they, and how did you handle any cravings you might have had?

The two hardest things to give up were white bread and processed cheese. A close third was white pasta. Growing up in an Italian household, pasta was a staple.

At the beginning, I would just give myself permission to eat as much of anything else I wanted that was a real food, until the craving went away. I would let myself do it even if I wasn't hungry, which I know goes against all of the conventional wisdom out there, but it worked for me. It's not a forever kind of thing, since the cravings lessen over time, and as your taste buds start to change, you start to crave the wholesome foods that are nourishing you from the inside out. It also helped once I learned how to make substitutes for these foods, but by then the cravings weren't as bad anyway, so I was able to enjoy them without comparing them to their processed counterparts.

Did you actually lose weight when you started eating real foods? If so, how would you explain the weight loss? How many pounds/ sizes did you lose?

I did lose weight when I started eating whole foods. In less than a year I lost 80 pounds.

Do you think that blogging and becoming part of a community of folks who also were working toward or had already made the change to a real-food/whole food diet helped you? If so, in what way?

I found that for me, especially at the beginning, it was invaluable to be on forums that were in line with the dietary choices I was making for myself (and later my whole family). It provided not only a sense of community and camaraderie, but also a level of accountability that I wouldn't have gotten at home on my own. It's not so much that any of the forums could make me do it if I didn't really want to. But for me, it was like a self-imposed obligation to not let them down, which would then guarantee not letting myself down. It also gave me the opportunity to ask questions and sometimes get answers from those who had been in the same place before me, plus help others who came after me.

Did your taste buds or palate change as a result of making the switch? If so, how so? Are there any real foods that you now find yourself wanting or craving?

My taste buds and palate did both change. My sense of taste has heightened to a point where I can actually pick out ingredients in a dish upon tasting it now. I wasn't able to do that before making the switch. It's like my taste buds were asleep from all of the abuse I had put them through and now they are thanking me for eating real foods by giving me this new gift, so to speak.

The real food I just can't seem to get enough of right now is sauerkraut. I have liked sauerkraut since I was a kid, but didn't have it all that often. However, for weeks now I've been eating it with almost every meal.

What would you suggest other parents do to make the transition to real foods for their kids?

Make it fun. Involve your kids. Nobody likes a dictator in or out of the kitchen. Teach kids about the foods they're eating so that they know what different foods do and don't do for their bodies. Changing your own diet is hard enough, so getting someone else to do it is even harder. You don't want to take a hard-line approach so much as do things to make it fun and appealing. If the kids are involved and having fun, they're that much more likely to try new things and enjoy the process, which leads to a longer lasting lifestyle and dietary change.

CHAPTER 12

Christine's Real-Food Cuisine

I hope I have convinced you by now that the road to lasting weight loss and better health leads not to the freezer case or fast food drive through, but to your very own kitchen. Replacing factory food and refined ingredients with real food does inevitably mean you are going to be doing more cooking, but it also means you'll know exactly what is in the meals you eat.

In this chapter, you'll find more than 100 recipes that will help you incorporate real foods into your menus, from easy breakfasts and lunches, to weeknight dinners and dishes that are perfect for entertaining—even fun cocktails and party nibbles. All are made with 100 percent real food, and each one is also 100 percent crowd-pleasingly delicious. Feel free to mix and match them with your own favorite recipes (made with real foods, of course). Just be sure you observe the basic nutrient guidelines for a Real-Food Weight Loss program: about 1,500 calories per day (2,000 for men) and to stabilize blood sugar, 20 to 25 grams of protein, 40 to 50 grams of carbohydrate, and 15 grams of fat per meal, and 10 to 15 grams of protein, 20 to 25 grams of carbs, and 10 grams of fat per snack serving. (See pages 117 to 119 for more on daily nutrient and calorie requirements.)

Because stable blood sugar levels are the heart of the Real-Food Weight Loss Diet, take care to have a PC or FC combo at every meal. Some of my recipes provide a PC Combo or FC Combo all on their own; others should be paired with another dish to create a healthful PC or FC combo. For example if you want to make a batch of the Lemony Blueberry Muffins for breakfast, keep in mind that you should consume the muffin with a lean protein source such as Greek yogurt or scrambled eggs. I've labeled all the recipes to make menu planning easier. You may also notice that some of these recipes are higher in fat than what you may be accustomed to eating on a diet plan; not to worry, though, the fats are all of the good-for-you variety. I have added notes at the bottom of some of the recipes to help inspire your taste buds and fine tune your weight loss. Lastly, there are a few recipes, such as the Coconut Water Kefir and Homemade Sauerkraut that are so low in calories I call them a "free food."

REAL-FOOD RECIPE KEY

🟢 = gluten free	For those who cannot tolerate gluten
🟢 = dairy free	For those who avoid dairy
PC = protein carb combo	These recipes are perfectly balanced
FC = fat carb combo	These recipes are perfectly balanced
PFC = protein carb fat	These recipes are a balance of all three nutrients
FF = fat friendly	These recipes are mainly friendly fats and should be combined with healthy carbohydrates
CC = carbohydrate concentrated	These recipes are high in healthy carbs and should be combined with a lean protein and/or a friendly fat
PP = protein powered	These recipes are high in protein and should be combined with healthy carbohydrates

Lemony Blueberry Muffins

MAKES 12 MUFFINS

Zsweet is an all-natural zero-calorie sweetener made from erythritol (an FDA-approved extract of the stevia plant) and natural flavors from made from botanical extracts. Dr. Andrew Weil and Dr. Nicholas Perricone endorse Zsweet, and that's good enough for me! It can be found at many natural foods stores and online; if you cannot find it, substitute the equivalent amount of xylitol.

2 cups whole wheat flour

½ cup Zsweet sweetener

1 teaspoon baking powder

½ teaspoon baking soda

½ teaspoon fine sea salt

¼ teaspoon ground cinnamon

⅛ teaspoon ground nutmeg

½ cup buttermilk

½ cup unsweetened organic applesauce

1 large egg

1 tablespoon grated lemon zest

1 cup blueberries

Preheat the oven to 400°F. Coat a 12-cup muffin pan with cooking spray or line with paper liners.

Whisk together the flour, Zsweet, baking powder, baking soda, sea salt, cinnamon, and nutmeg in a medium bowl. Whisk together the buttermilk, applesauce, egg, and lemon zest in a separate bowl. Add the flour mixture to the buttermilk mixture and stir with a large spoon just until combined (don't overmix). Gently fold in the blueberries.

Spoon the batter into the muffin cups and bake until a wooden pick inserted in the center comes out clean, about 20 minutes.

Cool the muffins in the pan on a rack.

Nutrition facts per muffin: 100 calories, 4 grams protein, 19 grams carbohydrates, 1 gram fat

PFC Hint: Have with Greek yogurt or eggs.

South of the Border Scramble

I like to use beef bacon because it's lower in fat than pork bacon, yet loaded with that yummy, smoky, bacon flavor. And yes this does use canned sauce, beans, and chiles, but because they are 99 percent all-natural ingredients, I consider them real foods and thus they get my thumbs up.

1 large egg

Splash of milk (any type that you desire)

1 teaspoon olive oil

Pinch of fine sea salt

Ground black pepper

1 tablespoon minced shallot

1 tablespoon chopped green chiles (canned is okay)

¼ cup canned black beans, rinsed and drained

1 slice uncured beef bacon

2 tablespoons canned enchilada sauce

1 tablespoon 0% or 2% Greek yogurt

1 teaspoon minced fresh cilantro (optional)

1 corn tortilla (6-inch)

Whisk together the egg, milk, sea salt, and pepper to taste. Set aside.

Heat ½ teaspoon of the oil in a small nonstick skillet over medium heat. Add the shallot and cook, stirring often, until softened, about 3 minutes. Add the green chiles and cook another 30 seconds. Add the egg mixture and cook, stirring occasionally, until the eggs are scrambled to your liking, 3 to 4 minutes. Add the black beans and stir to combine.

Meanwhile, heat the remaining ½ teaspoon oil in a small skillet over medium heat. Cook the beef bacon until crispy, about 3 minutes per side. Drain on paper towels.

Spoon the egg mixture onto a plate. Top with the enchilada sauce and yogurt. Sprinkle with the cilantro if desired. Serve with the tortilla and bacon.

Nutrition facts per serving: 342 calories, 16 grams protein, 29 grams carbohydrates, 19 grams fat

Petite Asparagus Frittatas

SERVES 4

If you don't have a sturdy muffin tin, no worries: I find that the aluminum muffin tins from the grocery store make perfectly baked mini frittatas.

½ pound asparagus

9 egg whites (preferably from cage free eggs)

3 eggs (preferably cage free)

2 tablespoons half-and-half

¼ cup shredded Romano cheese

1 tablespoon extra-virgin olive oil

1 small onion, diced

½ red bell pepper, cut into ½-inch strips

½ orange bell pepper, cut into ½-inch strips

Fine sea salt and ground black pepper

Preheat the oven to 375°F. Coat a 12-cup muffin tins pan with cooking spray.

Bring a medium pot of water to a boil. Add the asparagus and cook until tender, about 6 minutes. Drain and cool under cold running water. Cut into 1-inch pieces. Set aside.

Beat together the egg whites, whole eggs, half-and-half, and cheese in a medium bowl.

Heat 1 tablespoon of the oil in a large skillet over medium heat. Add the onion and bell peppers and cook until soft, 3 to 4 minutes. Add the asparagus and cook to heat through. Season with salt and pepper to taste.

Divide the vegetables among the muffin cups; they should be about half full. Ladle the egg mixture over the vegetables; do not fill the cups more than three-fourths full, as the eggs will puff up as they cook. Bake until a wooden pick inserted in the center of a frittata comes out clean, about 15 minutes.

Nutrition facts per serving (3 mini frittatas): 171 calories, 16 grams protein, 7 grams carbohydrates, 9 grams fat

PFC Hint: Have with a piece of toast.

Cremini-Mozza Quiche

SERVES 8

One Christmas morning, I got up early to make breakfast for my extended family. Taking in the sugar-loaded breakfast items all over the house, I immediately had a vision of the whole crew loaded up on sweets with spiked blood sugar and thought: Not on my watch! I found some zucchini and mushrooms left over from Christmas Eve dinner, pulled out some eggs, and the crustless quiche was born. It was a huge hit even with the little ones in our group. Make this for a holiday or any day!

1 tablespoon butter (preferably organic)

1 pound cremini mushrooms, coarsely chopped

3 teaspoons fresh thyme leaves

1 pound golden zucchini, cut into small dice

18 egg whites (about 2½ cups)

2 large eggs (preferably cage free)

1 cup half-and-half

1 teaspoon sea salt

1 teaspoon ground black pepper

¼ teaspoon hot sauce

1 cup grated part-skim mozzarella cheese

Preheat the oven to 375°F. Coat a 9-inch pie plate with cooking spray.

Melt the butter in a heavy medium skillet over medium heat. Add the mushrooms and 1 teaspoon of the thyme and cook until softened, 5 to 7 minutes. Add the squash and 1 teaspoon of the thyme. Cook until squash is just tender, about 5 minutes. Cool to room temperature and drain off any liquid.

Whisk together the egg whites, whole eggs, half-and-half, salt, pepper, and hot sauce in a bowl.

Spread the sautéed vegetables over the bottom of the pie plate and sprinkle with the cheese. Place the pie plate on a baking sheet and set it on a pulled-out oven rack. Pour the egg mixture over the vegetables, filling the pan completely (you may have some egg mixture left over). Sprinkle the remaining 1 teaspoon thyme over the top.

Bake until the quiche is golden and set in the center, about 35 minutes. Cool for at least 15 minutes on a rack before cutting into wedges and serving warm or at room temperature.

Nutrition facts per serving: 171 calories, 17 grams protein, 7 grams carbohydrates, 9 grams fat

PFC Hint: Serve with fresh fruit.

Canadian Sunrise Sandwich

SERVES 1

This is a delicious and healthy alternative to a fast-food breakfast sandwich, and it will take you more time to get to the nearest drive-thru than it would to make this tasty creation!

3 slices Canadian bacon (preferably nitrite and nitrate free)

1 slice reduced-fat smoked Gouda

1 large egg

Splash of milk or water

Fine sea salt and ground black pepper

2 slices whole wheat sourdough sandwich bread

1½ teaspoons whole grain mustard (or to taste)

Heat the Canadian bacon in a small skillet over medium heat for 1 minute, just to warm it through. Drain on a paper towel.

Whisk together the egg, milk or water, and salt and pepper to taste in a small bowl.

Coat the same skillet with cooking spray and heat over medium heat. Add the egg mixture and stir occasionally with a wooden spoon until scrambled, 3 to 4 minutes depending on your preference.

To assemble the sandwich, spread both slices of bread with the mustard. Layer the gouda, egg, and bacon on one slice. Close the sandwich and place in a panini press and heat until the bread is toasted and the cheese is melted, 4 to 5 minutes. (If you do not have a panini press, simply toast the bread first, then assemble the sandwich.)

Nutrition facts per serving: 369 calories, 24 grams protein, 34 grams carbohydrates, 12 grams fat

Rustic German Apple Pancake

SERVES 6

For years I avoided pancakes because foods that are extremely high in carbohydrates and low in protein can cause blood sugar spikes and dips. Compared to the average everyday pancake, this German apple pancake recipe is loaded with healthy protein and fiber. Best of all it's a guaranteed crowd pleaser because of its fluffy texture and beautiful appearance. The apple slices make it look like it came straight out of a German neighborhood cafe.

½ cup whole wheat flour

½ teaspoon baking powder

¼ cup ground flaxseed meal

1 tablespoon coconut palm sugar or organic cane sugar

⅛ teaspoon fine sea salt

⅛ teaspoon plus 1 teaspoon ground cinnamon

1 cup egg whites (from about 7 eggs, preferably cage free)

1 cup coconut milk

2 tablespoons coconut oil, melted

1 teaspoon pure vanilla extract

¼ cup Zsweet

3 green apples, unpeeled, halved and thinly sliced

1 tablespoon confectioners' sugar

Whisk together the flour, baking powder, flax meal, sugar, salt, and ⅛ teaspoon of the cinnamon in a medium bowl.

Beat together the egg whites, coconut milk, coconut oil, and vanilla in a small bowl. Add to the flour mixture and whisk well until combined. Let stand for 30 minutes.

Preheat the oven to 425°F. Coat the bottom and sides of a 10-inch ovenproof skillet with cooking spray. Combine the Zsweet and remaining 1 teaspoon cinnamon in a small bowl; sprinkle half of the mixture evenly over bottom and sides of the pan. Arrange the apple slices in the pan in a single layer, in a spoke pattern. Sprinkle with the remaining cinnamon mixture. Cook over medium heat undisturbed until the mixture bubbles, about 8 minutes.

Carefully pour the batter evenly over the apple slices. Transfer to the oven, being careful not to spill the batter, and bake for 15 minutes. Reduce the oven temperature to 375°F and bake until the center is set, about 13 minutes.

Cool for 5 minutes, then gently loosen the pancake from the skillet with a spatula and slide onto a serving platter. Sift the confectioners' sugar over the top. Cut into 6 wedges and serve warm.

Nutrition facts per wedge: 270 calories, 8 grams protein, 29 grams carbohydrates, 15 grams fat (all good fats!)

Bangin' Banana Bread

MAKES 16 SLICES

2 ripe bananas, mashed

½ cup unsweetened organic applesauce

2 large eggs (preferably cage free)

⅓ cup 0% or 2% Greek yogurt

½ cup Zsweet

½ cup organic brown sugar

1 cup whole wheat flour

¼ cup ground flaxseed meal

1 teaspoon fine sea salt

¾ teaspoon baking soda

½ teaspoon ground cinnamon

Preheat the oven to 350°F. Coat a 9 x 5-inch loaf pan with cooking spray.

With an electric mixer on medium speed, beat the bananas, applesauce, eggs, and yogurt in a large bowl. Beat in the Zsweet and brown sugar until combined.

Whisk together the flour, flax meal, salt, baking soda, and cinnamon in a medium bowl. Add the flour mixture to the banana mixture and beat until blended.

Pour the batter into the loaf pan and bake until a wooden pick inserted in the center comes out clean, 50 to 55 minutes. Cool in the pan for 10 minutes then turn out onto a rack to cool completely. Cut into ½-inch slices.

Nutrition facts per ½-inch slice: 93 calories, 18 grams carbohydrates, 2 grams protein, 2 grams fat

PFC Hint: Have with Greek yogurt or eggs.

Fresh Baked Granola

MAKES 8 GENEROUS CUPS

This granola is a great alternative to packaged cereal. I boost its antioxidant quotient by adding dried goji berries, but you can use any dried fruit you prefer. Serve with fresh fruit and milk; coconut milk tastes great with this granola.

3 cups old-fashioned rolled oats

1½ cups unsweetened shredded coconut

½ cup unsweetened wheat germ

1 cup unsalted hulled sunflower seeds

¼ cup sesame seeds

½ cup raw organic honey

¼ cup coconut oil, melted

1 cup slivered almonds

½ cup goji berries

Position a rack in the center of the oven and preheat to 225°F. Coat a large rimmed baking sheet with cooking spray.

Toss together the oats, shredded coconut, wheat germ, sunflower seeds, and sesame seeds in an extra large bowl.

Stir together the honey and coconut oil in a small bowl. Drizzle over the dry ingredients and mix well. Add ½ cup cold water a little at a time, stirring well after each addition, until the mixture is crumbly. Pour the mixture onto the baking sheet and spread evenly to the edges of the pan.

Bake for 1 hour 30 minutes, stirring every 15 minutes. Add the almonds and bake until the mixture is thoroughly dry and golden brown, about 30 minutes.

Remove from the oven, mix in the goji berries, and cool on the baking sheet. When completely cool, transfer the granola to a tightly covered container or resealable plastic bag and store in the refrigerator.

Nutrition facts per ¼ cup: 140 calories, 3 grams protein, 12 grams carbohydrates, 9 grams fat

PFC Hint: Have with soy or coconut milk.

Jeweled Steel-Cut Oats

SERVES 4

Most people feel they don't have the time for steel-cut oats because they take about 20 minutes longer to cook than regular oats. However, soaking the oats overnight in water with an acid—such as vinegar, lemon juice, or kefir—reduces the cooking time tremendously. And once you have done this a few times, it becomes second nature. The best ratio is 1½ cups water plus 1 tablespoon of an acid for each ½ cup of uncooked oats. (Alternatively, you can simply follow package directions and endure the extra cooking time.)

1 cup steel-cut oats

2 tablespoons fresh lemon juice

¼ teaspoon fine sea salt

2 dashes ground cinnamon

2 tablespoons crushed walnuts

½ cup blueberries

½ cup pitted cherries

½ cup soymilk or light coconut milk

Combine the oats and lemon juice with 3 cups water in a bowl. Let soak overnight.

Drain the water from the oats. Bring 2 cups fresh water to a boil in a medium pot. Add the oats, salt, and cinnamon. Stir well, reduce the heat to low, and simmer, stirring occasionally, until soft, about 10 minutes.

Spoon the oatmeal into serving bowls, and top with the walnuts, blueberries, cherries, and soy or coconut milk.

Nutrition facts per ½-cup serving: 200 calories, 9 grams protein, 34 grams carbohydrates, 5 grams fat

PFC Hint: Have with coconut milk for an FC combo.

Coconut Water Kefir

MAKES 2 QUARTS

This wonderful fermented drink has helped my clients (and me!) improve their digestion, reduce bloating, and feel more energized. This recipe yields quite a few servings because it's most efficient to make the coconut water kefir in large quantities so that you don't have to repeat the recipe for at least a week. (Use the leftover coconut meat for the coconut kefir yogurt recipe that follows.) I like to make up large batches on Sundays. Kefir grains (which are also called Japanese water crystals) are tiny crystal-like pieces that are actually healthy living bacteria. When you add them to liquid they begin to release enzymes that permeate whatever substance they are living in. In water, milk, ice cream, or yogurt, they help improve immunity, digestion, and nutrient absorption, which is helpful during the weight loss process. If you don't have a local source for kefir grains you can buy them online at www.happyherbalist.com/japanesewatercrystals.aspx).

1 quart fresh coconut water (from young Thai coconuts; see Note) or store-bought coconut water

1 tablespoon kefir grains

Strain the coconut water through a sieve into a large jar with a tight-fitting lid. Add the kefir grains, screw on the cover, and let sit at room temperature for 1 day. Strain out the grains, cover the coconut water kefir, and store in the refrigerator for up to 4 weeks.

Note: To split a young Thai coconut, set the coconut on a cutting board flat side down. With the bottom corner of the blade of a chef's knife (just above the handle), whack the coconut just underneath the top of the coconut where it begins to round, hacking into it downward with the blade. Turn the coconut and hit it again two more times to make three holes through the top of the coconut in a triangle formation. Insert the bottom edge of the knife into one of the holes, wiggle the knife and slowly continue to wedge it into the coconut and the top will literally pop off in a perfect circular shape. Puff! You can then easily pour the coconut water out into a jar. Scoop the coconut meat out using a small offset spatula and set it aside to use in the coconut kefir yogurt recipe.

Nutrition facts per ¼-cup serving: 20 calories, 1 gram protein, 4 grams carbohydrates, 0 grams fat

Free Food: This is so low in calories you can consider 2 servings per day free.

Coconut "Faux"gurt

MAKES 14 CUPS

Coconuts, coconut oil, and coconut milk have gotten a bad rap from a 1950s study that was based on hydrogenated coconut oil. Although coconut oil is about 87 percent saturated fat, in its unrefined, virgin state, it is actually beneficial, thanks largely to its lauric acid content. Lauric acid has potent antiviral and antibacterial properties. Recent studies have suggested coconut oil might have applications for lowering viral levels in HIV-AIDS patients, as well as fighting yeast and fungal infections, and other viruses such as herpes simplex and influenza.

I can attest to the antiviral properties of coconut oil. For years I have suffered from stress-related cold sore breakouts on my face. About 11 months ago, I started a preventive regimen of coconut oil, adding a tablespoon to my tea every morning and a tablespoon to a glass of warm water each night before bed. When I recently went through a very stressful divorce, move, and complete life restructure, I did not get one cold sore. Additionally, I no longer have any premenstrual symptoms and I credit much of this to adding coconut oil to my diet.

1 vanilla bean, split

Meat from 6 young Thai coconuts

1 cup coconut kefir (homemade or store-bought)

3 tablespoons Zsweet or granulated stevia

Shaved dark chocolate (70% cacao)

Fresh mint leaves, for garnish

Working in 2 batches, scrape half of the vanilla seeds into a blender and add half the coconut meat, coconut kefir, and Zsweet. Blend until the mixture is thick and smooth, about 3 minutes. Transfer to a pitcher and repeat with the remaining vanilla seeds, coconut meat, kefir, and sweetener. Store in a covered container in the refrigerator for up to 7 days. Serve chilled in a tall glass garnished with shaved dark chocolate and a mint leaf.

Nutrition facts per 1-cup serving: 130 calories, 9 grams protein, 21 grams carbohydrates, 5 grams fat

Razzy Peach Parfait

SERVES 1

This parfait also works as a fantastic lunch, snack, or dinner for times when you don't feeling like cooking.

6 ounces 0% or 2% Greek yogurt

1 tablespoon raw organic honey

1 tablespoon unsalted toasted hulled pumpkin seeds (pepitas)

¼ cup raspberries

1 peach, diced

Fine sea salt

Make layers in a tall parfait glass in this order: Greek yogurt, honey, pumpkin seeds, raspberries, peaches. Repeat the layering until you reach the top of the glass and all the ingredients have been used. Alternatively, combine the ingredients in a medium bowl, mix well, and spoon into a serving dish.

Nutrition facts per serving: 341 calories, 24 grams protein, 48 grams carbohydrates, 9 grams fat

Açaí Superfood Smoothie

SERVES 1

This smoothie has a wonderful balance of natural sugars, monounsaturated fats (good for you), and protein to keep you feeling full. Not all protein powders are created equal! You need to read the labels (see page 117 for information on becoming a "label detective") or just use Jay Robb's brand of egg white protein, which is a Real-Food Diet–approved protein source in my opinion.

Although açaí is often touted as a weight loss aid, there are very few human studies to support such claims. But I like açaí for its delicious tart and slightly sweet flavor and its kickbutt antioxidant power. The açaí berry has approximately ten times the antioxidants of grapes and twice the antioxidants of blueberries, as well as omega-3s. It's also high in living enzymes and is a natural anti-inflammatory. According to traditional Chinese medicine it helps diminish candida-causing yeast in the body. Most exciting, many folks claim that açaí helps improve sexual performance . . . hubba hubba!

1 cup frozen blueberries

½ cup frozen strawberries

1 cup light coconut milk

¼ cup açaí berry juice

1 scoop (1 ounce) high-quality protein powder (such as Jay Robb's egg white protein)

10 ice cubes

Combine all the ingredients in a blender and puree until smooth.

Nutrition facts per serving: 384 calories, 26 grams protein, 42 grams carbohydrates, 13 grams fat (all good fats!)

Christine's Fave Coconut Smoothie

SERVES 1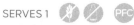

The burst of tropical flavors in this smoothie will transport you to an exotic beach. And if you stick to my plan you will feel great in a bikini on that beach!

1 cup light coconut milk, chilled

1 large banana

2 tablespoons ground flaxseed meal

1 scoop (1 ounce) high-quality protein powder (such as Jay Robb's egg white protein)

10 ice cubes

Combine all the ingredients in a blender and puree until smooth.

Nutrition facts per serving: 369 calories, 28 grams protein, 36 grams carbohydrates, 17 grams fat (all good fats!)

Espresso Smoothie

SERVES 1

The tradition of starting each morning with the smell and taste of a freshly brewed espresso is one of the many things I love about my Italian heritage. I get that flavor—and the protein and carbohydrates I need to make it a meal—from this smoothie. Bellissimo!

1 cup light coconut milk, chilled

2 tablespoons ground flaxseed meal

1 shot brewed espresso (or really strong coffee), chilled

1 scoop (1 ounce) high-quality protein powder (such as Jay Robb's egg white protein)

10 ice cubes

Combine all the ingredients in a blender and puree until smooth.

Nutrition facts per serving: 397 calories, 28 grams protein, 36 grams carbohydrates, 17 grams fat (all good fats!)

Georgia Peach Smoothie

SERVES 1

I grew up eating both pomegranates and peaches (which were grown on my grandparents' farm) and have always loved those flavors. Little did I know how good they were for me. They are even better together—double bonus!

1 cup light coconut milk, chilled

1 tablespoon ground flaxseed meal

½ cup pomegranate seeds

1 peach, diced

1 scoop (1 ounce) high quality protein powder (such as Jay Robb's egg white protein)

10 ice cubes

Combine all the ingredients in a blender and puree until smooth.

Nutrition facts per serving: 369 calories, 27 grams protein, 33 grams carbohydrates, 15 grams fat (all good fats!)

Fizzie Fruit Smoothie

SERVES 1

Make sure your juice is 100 percent juice and not one of those sugar-sweetened, fruit-flavored beverages claiming to be juice! If you cannot find açaí berry juice, blueberry, pomegranate, or cherry juice is a good substitute.

1 cup Coconut Water Kefir (page 204)

1 tablespoon coconut oil, melted

½ cup açaí berry juice (or your favorite naturally sweetened pure fruit juice)

1 cup frozen blueberries

1 scoop high-quality protein powder (such as Jay Robb's egg white protein)

10 ice cubes

Combine all the ingredients in a blender and puree until smooth.

Nutrition facts per serving: 360 calories, 26 grams protein, 33 grams carbohydrates, 15 grams fat (all good fats!)

Butternut Sage Soup

SERVES 8

Each fall when there is a crisp chill in the air, all I want is something that will warm me from the inside out. For times like those, this soup hits the spot. I sometimes garnish the soup with a bit of crumbled organic goat cheese; however this will increase the fat content of the soup, so don't overdo it.

1 slice uncured beef bacon, diced

2 tablespoons extra-virgin olive oil

1 medium onion, diced

3 garlic cloves, minced

1 large butternut squash (about 2¼ pounds), peeled and cubed

4 cups chicken stock

2 teaspoons minced chipotle chiles in adobo

2 cups white sweet corn kernels (fresh or frozen, thawed)

8 teaspoons 0% or 2% Greek yogurt

1 teaspoon fine sea salt

½ teaspoon ground black pepper

2 sprigs fresh sage, chopped

Cook the bacon in a large soup pot over medium-high heat until extra crisp, about 5 minutes. Use a slotted spoon to transfer the bacon bits to a paper towel–lined plate, leaving any rendered fat in the pan.

Add the oil, onion, and garlic to the pot and cook until the onions are translucent, 4 to 5 minutes. Add the squash, stock, and chipotles and bring to a boil. Reduce the heat to medium and cook at a gentle boil, stirring occasionally, until the squash is soft, about 20 minutes. Add the corn and cook for 5 minutes.

Using a hand blender or regular blender, puree the soup, leaving some chunks or to your desired consistency. Garnish each serving with 1 teaspoon Greek yogurt, a few bacon bits, and some sage.

Nutrition facts per 1½-cup serving: 190 calories, 6 grams protein, 30 grams of carbohydrates, 6 grams fat

PFC Hint: Have with lean protein such as grilled chicken or fish.

Farmers' Market "Tortilla" Soup

SERVES 6

I love tortilla soup because of the heat and flavor the Mexican spices contribute, and it's even better with all these yummy, delicious veggies.

1 pound boneless, skinless chicken breasts, cut into 1-inch chunks

1½ teaspoons fine sea salt

1 teaspoon cumin seeds

1 teaspoon chili powder

1 teaspoon dried oregano

1 teaspoon cayenne pepper

1 teaspoon red pepper flakes

1 teaspoon fresh cracked black pepper

3 teaspoons extra-virgin olive oil

1 large onion, diced

3 garlic cloves, minced

2 celery ribs, diced

2 carrots, diced

20 grape tomatoes, halved

1 can (28 ounces) crushed tomatoes (preferably San Marzano)

4 cups chicken stock

½ cup corn kernels, thawed frozen or scraped from 1 grilled or boiled ear

¼ bunch cilantro, chopped (optional)

1 bunch scallions, chopped

¼ cup 0% or 2% Greek yogurt

1 to 2 limes, cut into wedges

Place the chicken in a medium bowl and sprinkle with 1 teaspoon of the salt and ½ teaspoon each of the cumin, chili powder, oregano, cayenne pepper, red pepper flakes, and cracked black pepper. Drizzle with 1½ teaspoons of the oil and toss to coat. Cover the bowl with plastic wrap and let marinate in the refrigerator for at least 30 minutes while you prepare the soup.

Heat the remaining 1½ teaspoons oil in a large soup pot or Dutch oven over medium heat. Add the onions, half the garlic, and the remaining ½ teaspoon each cumin, chili powder, oregano, cayenne, red pepper flakes, sea salt, and cracked black pepper. Cook until the onions are soft and translucent, about 5 minutes.

Add the celery, carrots, and grape tomatoes and cook for 5 minutes. Add the canned tomatoes, reduce the heat to low, and cook, stirring frequently, until the mixture thickens and takes on a reddish orange color, 10 to 15 minutes.

Stir in the stock and bring to a gentle boil over medium-high heat. Once the soup is boiling, reduce the heat to medium-low and simmer for 15 minutes.

Add the corn and marinated chicken and cook until the chicken is cooked through, about 10 minutes. Serve garnished with the cilantro (if using), scallions, and a dollop of Greek yogurt with lime wedges on the side.

Nutrition facts per 2¼-cup serving: 230 calories, 25 grams protein, 23 grams carbohydrates, 5 grams fat

Italian Lentil Soup

SERVES 8

Lentils are a great source of protein and taste amazing in this soup, which is similar to the one my grandmother Rosemary made often on our family ranch in Gilroy, California. She added mini pasta shells, the kind used in macaroni salad. This is major comfort food for me. . . . I sincerely hope you enjoy it as much as my family and I have. Swap the chicken stock for vegetable stock to make this a vegetarian option. I like to soak the lentils overnight, but if you don't have time, soak them for 1 hour and use an additional 2 to 3 cups of water to simmer the soup.

1 pound lentils

¼ cup extra-virgin olive oil

1 teaspoon dried oregano

1 large onion, diced

2 garlic cloves, minced

8 cups low-sodium chicken stock

1 can (14.5 ounces) diced tomatoes

1 can (15 ounces) tomato sauce

Fine sea salt and ground black pepper

3 tablespoons minced fresh oregano (optional)

3 tablespoons 0% or 2% Greek yogurt (optional)

Cover the lentils with water and soak overnight. Drain the lentils and set aside.

Heat the oil in a medium or large pot (at least 6 quarts) over medium heat. Add the dried oregano, onion, and garlic and cook, stirring frequently, for 5 minutes. Add the stock, 8 cups of water (increase the water to 10 to 11 cups if the lentils were not soaked overnight), the tomatoes and tomato sauce. Bring to a gentle boil and cook for several minutes. Add the lentils, return to a gentle boil and cook until the lentils are very tender, about 1 hour. Season with salt and pepper to taste.

Garnish each serving with fresh oregano and a dab of Greek yogurt if desired.

Nutrition facts per 1½-cup serving: 330 calories, 19 grams protein, 42 grams carbohydrates, 8 grams fat

Quick Tomato Soup

SERVES 8

One cold winter day I was craving tomato soup with a grilled cheese sandwich. (BTW, I have a great grilled cheese recipe in my first book, Skinny Chicks Don't Eat Salads.*) Unfortunately, I did not have any fresh tomatoes on hand that I could roast so I used some organic canned diced tomatoes instead. The soup tasted fabulous and was incredibly easy to make. That's what real food in real life is all about; even when we don't have fresh ingredients we can still make healthy, great tasting real food!*

1 tablespoon extra-virgin olive oil

4 garlic cloves, minced

¼ teaspoon cayenne pepper

¼ teaspoon red pepper flakes

1 medium white onion, chopped

2 celery ribs, diced

2 carrots, diced

2 cups chicken stock

2 cans (15 ounces each) tomato sauce

1 can (15 ounces) cannellini beans (white kidney beans), rinsed and drained

Fine sea salt and ground black pepper

Heat the oil into a large soup pot over medium heat. Add the garlic, cayenne, and pepper flakes and cook for 1 minute. Add the onion, celery and carrots and cook until the onion is translucent, about 7 minutes. Add the stock and tomato sauce, bring to a gentle boil and cook, stirring occasionally, for 5 minutes. Add the beans and simmer for 5 minutes. Season with sea salt and pepper to taste.

Nutrition facts per 1½-cup serving: 248 calories, 12 grams protein, 38 grams carbohydrates, 6 grams fat

PFC Hint: Have with a grilled cheese sandwich made with low fat, real-food cheese.

Arugula and Beet Salad

SERVES 4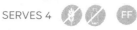

The sweetness of the beets with the peppery arugula is a wonderful palate pleaser. Sometimes I add goat cheese to this salad, and it's amazing! If you don't have time to roast the beets, you can often find vacuum-packed roasted beets in the produce sections of better supermarkets.

2 medium beets

4 cups arugula

2 tablespoons plus 1 teaspoon extra-virgin olive oil

1 tablespoon balsamic vinegar

Fine sea salt and cracked black pepper

Preheat the oven to 425°F. Trim the stems off the beets and lightly scrub with a vegetable brush. Wrap in foil and roast until tender, about 45 minutes. When cool enough to handle, peel the beets and cut into ½-inch cubes— you should have about 1 cup. Chill to at least room temperature before making the salad. (You can also roast the beets up to 2 days ahead of time.) Toss the arugula and beets in a large bowl. Whisk together the oil and vinegar in a small bowl until emulsified. Add a pinch of salt and cracked pepper to the dressing. Pour the dressing over the salad and toss well.

Nutrition facts per serving: 90 calories, 1 gram protein, 5 grams carbohydrates, 7 grams fat

PFC Hint: Serve alongside fish and rice or any balanced PC combo.

Avocado-Tomato Salad

SERVES 4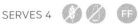

Like ebony and ivory, this salad is in perfect harmony, with the richness of the avocado balancing the acidity of the tomatoes! Best of all, the avocados are so creamy that you don't need to add any oil to make this salad yummy.

2 Hass avocados, diced

½ pint cherry tomatoes

1 tablespoon fresh lemon juice

¼ teaspoon fine sea salt

⅛ teaspoon ground black pepper

Combine all the ingredients in a salad bowl and toss gently to coat.

Nutrition facts per ½-cup serving: 170 calories, 3 grams protein, 10 grams carbohydrates, 15 grams fat (all good fats!)

PFC Hint: Serve with hard-cooked eggs and fresh fruit.

Cucumber Salad with Yuzu and Sesame

SERVES 5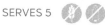

Yuzu is a lovely citrus fruit from East Asia. It is a sour mandarin hybrid and tastes somewhat like a lemony orange. You can find it at most Asian markets. Serve this salad alongside any of my Asian mains; the refreshing flavors balance well with the richness of a dish like the Mongolian Beef (page 235).

2 cucumbers, very thinly sliced

1 tablespoon toasted sesame seeds

1 tablespoon rice vinegar

2 teaspoons yuzu juice (if you cannot find yuzu, use lemon juice)

Fine sea salt and ground black pepper

Combine the cucumbers, sesame seeds, vinegar, and yuzu juice in a medium bowl and toss lightly. Season with salt and pepper to taste.

Nutrition facts per ½-cup serving: 70 calories, 2 gram protein, 4 grams carbohydrates, 5 grams fat

PFC Hint: Almost a free food, serve with any balanced meal.

Spicy Tuna Pokē

SERVES 4

Pokē is a Hawaiian raw fish salad, somewhat like Mexican ceviche. There are many ways it can be prepared. If you are ever in Hawaii, I highly recommend tasting the various pokēs the local eateries have to offer. My version is so authentic you will feel as if you are in the islands. Aloha!

½ pound sashimi-grade ahi tuna, cut into ½-inch cubes

½ small sweet onion, cut into matchsticks

2 scallions, thinly sliced

1 garlic clove, minced

1 teaspoon grated fresh ginger

3 tablespoons tamari or soy sauce

½ teaspoon toasted sesame oil

½ teaspoon Sriracha sauce (Thai chili sauce)

¼ teaspoon Chinese chili oil

½ teaspoon fine sea salt

¼ teaspoon red pepper flakes

1 tablespoon black sesame seeds

Combine all the ingredients in a medium bowl and toss well. Cover with plastic wrap and refrigerate for 1 hour. Serve chilled.

Nutrition facts per 4-ounce serving: 120 calories, 16 grams protein, 7 grams carbohydrates, 3 grams fat

Tuscan Kale Toss

SERVES 8

Cannellini beans give a basic Tuscan kale salad a real protein boost, and cherry tomatoes add a hint of sweetness to this salty, citrus-y dish. And with 7 grams of monounsaturated fatty acids, this salad will help burn belly fat!! Buon appetito!

1 bunch kale

1 garlic clove, minced

Fine sea salt

¼ cup grated Parmesan cheese

¼ cup extra-virgin olive oil

Juice of 1 lemon

¼ teaspoon red pepper flakes

¼ teaspoon anchovy paste

Cracked black pepper

½ cup canned cannellini beans (white kidney beans), rinsed and drained

½ cup halved cherry tomatoes

½ cup Homemade Croutons (opposite), crumbled

Wash the kale and tear out the stems. Cut the leaves into ¾-inch-wide ribbons and set aside in a large salad bowl.

Using a mortar and pestle or the back of a spoon, mash the garlic with ¼ teaspoon salt until it becomes a paste. Transfer to a bowl and add the cheese, oil, lemon juice, red pepper flakes, and anchovy paste. Whisk to combine all ingredients well. Add more salt and cracked pepper to taste.

Pour the dressing on the kale and toss well (this dressing is quite thick). Let sit for 5 minutes so that the lemon juice can begin to soften the kale.

Add the beans, tomatoes, and croutons and give the salad one more thorough toss.

Nutrition facts per serving: 180 calories, 6 grams protein, 16 grams carbohydrates, 11 grams fat

PFC Hint: This yummy salad is PFC but you can add another small portion of a PC combo such as chicken and baby potatoes.

Homemade Croutons

MAKES ABOUT 2 CUPS

These croutons are so easy to make and if you have any day-old bread in your breadbox this is always a great way to put it to use.

4 slices whole wheat sourdough bread, cut into 1-inch squares

1 tablespoon extra-virgin olive oil

1 tablespoon grated Parmesan cheese

1 garlic clove, minced

½ teaspoon dried oregano

½ teaspoon fine sea salt

½ teaspoon ground black pepper

Preheat the oven to 325°F. Toss together the bread, oil, cheese, garlic, oregano, salt, and pepper in a bowl, coating evenly. Spread on a baking sheet in a single layer. Bake, turning with a spatula every 10 minutes, until browned and crisp, 20 to 30 minutes. Cool on the baking sheet for 10 minutes. Store the cooled croutons in an airtight container for up to 2 weeks.

Nutrition facts per ¼-cup serving: 60 calories, 2 grams protein, 7 grams carbohydrates, 3 grams fat

Asian Quinoa Salad

SERVES 4

Serve this along with my Spicy Tuna Pokē (page 219) for a perfect PC combo.

½ cup quinoa

½ cup diced red bell pepper

½ cup thinly sliced scallions

½ cup diced cucumber

3 tablespoons fresh lime juice

1 tablespoon olive oil

1 teaspoon agave nectar

¼ teaspoon fine sea salt

¼ teaspoon ground black pepper

1 tablespoon black sesame seeds

¼ cup fresh cilantro leaves, coarsely chopped

Combine the quinoa and ½ cup water in a medium saucepan and bring to a boil over high heat. Cover, reduce to a simmer, and cook until the liquid is absorbed, about 15 minutes. Spoon the quinoa into a bowl and fluff with a fork. Add the bell pepper, scallions, and cucumber and toss to combine.

Whisk together the lime juice, olive oil, agave, salt, and black pepper in a small bowl. Add to quinoa mixture and toss well. Top with the sesame seeds and cilantro.

Nutrition facts per ⅔-cup serving: 238 calories, 6 grams protein, 35 grams carbohydrates, 9 grams fat

PFC Hint: Have with any lean protein.

Autumn Harvest Salad

SERVES 6

I often serve this salad at Passages Malibu because the clients and staff love it; it's our most popular salad by far. It's loaded with the sweet-tart taste of the dried cranberries layered with the tang of rice vinegar and the saltiness of soy sauce. Either way, it's always a joy to serve a dish that everybody loves.

DRESSING

2 tablespoons rice vinegar

1 tablespoon raw organic honey

1 teaspoon soy sauce

¼ cup extra-virgin olive oil

Fine sea salt and ground black pepper

SALAD

3 cups vegetable stock

1 cup brown rice

½ cup wild rice

1 celery rib, thinly sliced

½ cup dried cranberries

½ cup chopped walnuts

5 cups spring greens mix, baby spinach, or watercress

2 boneless, skinless chicken breasts, grilled and diced

2 ounces goat cheese, cut into small cubes

To make the dressing: Whisk together the vinegar, honey, soy sauce, and oil. Season with salt and pepper to taste.

To make the salad: Bring the broth to a boil in a medium pot. Add the brown rice and wild rice, reduce to a simmer, cover, and cook until the broth is absorbed and the rice is tender, about 50 minutes. Remove from the heat and let stand for 10 minutes. Fluff with a fork, turn out into a large bowl, and cool to room temperature.

Add the celery, cranberries, and walnuts to the rice mixture. Add the dressing and toss to combine.

Toss the greens with the rice mixture and serve topped with the chicken and cheese.

Nutrition facts per serving: 310 calories, 13 grams protein, 25 grams carbohydrates, 18 grams fat

Greek Isles Salad

SERVES 4

For the past two summers I've been lucky enough to vacation on the amazing Greek islands of Santorini and Mykonos. One dish I found myself eating every day was a delicious salad with the amazing flavors of local oregano, olive oil, cucumbers, and tomatoes. To relive that experience, I had to make a recipe that would satisfy my craving for those Greek-island flavors. This salad hits the spot every time!

DRESSING

⅓ cup extra-virgin olive oil

¼ cup red wine vinegar

1 tablespoon chopped fresh oregano

1 garlic clove, minced

2 teaspoons kosher salt

1 teaspoon ground black pepper

SALAD

2 heads romaine lettuce, torn into bite-size pieces

3 large heirloom tomatoes, seeded and coarsely chopped

1 red onion, thinly sliced

1 large cucumber, unpeeled, cut into rounds

¼ pound Kalamata olives, pitted and chopped

¼ pound cooked shrimp (grilled or boiled)

3 ounces feta cheese, crumbled

To make the dressing: Whisk together the oil, vinegar, oregano, garlic, salt, and pepper and whisk until thickened, about 1 minute.

To assemble the salad: Place the romaine in a large salad bowl and add the tomatoes, onion, cucumber, olives, and shrimp. Pour the dressing over all, toss to combine, and sprinkle with the feta. Serve immediately.

Nutrition facts per serving: 287 calories, 13 grams protein, 15 grams carbohydrates, 20 grams fat (mostly good fats!)

Spiced-Up Egg Salad

SERVES 1

Poor eggs... they get such a bad rap though they are actually quite good for you. I'm addicted to hard-cooked eggs (I eat one almost every day). When you can, choose organic, cage free, omega-3 eggs. Compared to conventionally pro-duced eggs, they have one-third less cholesterol, one-fourth less saturated fat, two-thirds more vitamin A, two times more omega-3 fatty acids, and three times more vitamins—practically a whole different food! This egg salad is very versa-tile: You can serve it on whole wheat toast, cucumber slices, celery, lettuce cups, or rice crackers.

2 hard-cooked eggs (preferably cage free), peeled and diced

1 celery rib, diced

1 tablespoon mayonnaise

¼ teaspoon Sriracha sauce (Thai chili sauce)

¼ teaspoon seeded, minced jalapeño chile pepper

⅛ teaspoon fine sea salt

⅛ teaspoon ground black pepper

Combine all the ingredients in a bowl and mix well.

Nutrition facts per serving: 180 calories, 12 grams protein, 5 grams carbohydrates, 12 grams fat

PFC Hint: Add a slice of Ezekiel bread or a piece of fruit.

Homemade Sauerkraut

MAKES 4 QUARTS

It's not hard to make your own sauerkraut and you'll be knocked out by how good it tastes. To ferment the sauerkraut safely it must remain in an anaerobic state (without oxygen). This is accomplished by keeping the cabbage and vegetables completely submerged in a salty brine, with a weight on top to keep the solids covered in liquid. You can use a ceramic crock, glass bowl, or food-grade bucket topped by a plate that fits inside the container you are using. You'll also need a weight for holding down the plate (I use my marble mortar because it's very heavy) and a dish cloth to cover the container as the sauerkraut ferments.

2 heads red cabbage

1 yellow bell pepper, diced

2 jalapeño chile peppers, seeded and minced

2 garlic cloves, minced

3 tablespoons fine sea salt

Using the slicing blade on a food processor, shred the cabbage in long pieces. If you do not have a food processor, thinly slice the cabbage with a chef's knife.

Toss together the cabbage, bell pepper, jalapeños, and garlic in a large bowl. Sprinkle with the salt and toss again. Transfer the cabbage mixture to the crock. Using your fists or a tamper, punch down the cabbage mixture until the vegetables begin to release their liquid. When the liquid from the cabbage mixture covers the cabbage, you are done. If the cabbage doesn't release enough liquid, add a brine of 1 tablespoon of salt to 1 cup of water.

Place a plate on the top of the cabbage and place a heavy weight on the plate to keep the vegetables fully submerged in the brine.

Cover with a dish towel and let the sauerkraut ferment for 7 days. Tamp down the sauerkraut several times during the first few hours of fermentation. This process releases a distinctive odor, so it is best to ferment your sauerkraut in the basement or a noncommon area in your home.

Nutrition facts per ½-cup serving: 25 calories, 1 gram protein, 6 grams carbohydrates, 0 grams fat

Free Food: It's because low in calories but it's only free if you have 2 servings or less!

Cilantro Chili Lime Dressing

MAKES ABOUT ½ CUP

My goal is to never waste anything in the kitchen! One evening when I was juicing limes to marinate some fish I found I had an extra lime left over. Of course I could not throw away that zesty green jewel, so I pulled out some Asian condiments and pretty soon I had a brand new dressing.

¼ cup vegetable oil

Juice of 1 lime

2 tablespoons rice vinegar

1 teaspoon soy sauce

1 teaspoon Sriracha sauce (Thai chili sauce)

1 teaspoon toasted sesame oil

1 teaspoon sesame seeds

¼ cup chopped fresh cilantro

Whisk all the ingredients together.

Nutrition facts per 1 tablespoon: 110 calories, 0 grams protein, 0 grams carbohydrates, 12 grams fat (all good fats!)

Tango Chimichurri

MAKES 1 CUP

I don't know about you but I love a good chimichurri on grilled meat or vegetables. One night my dear friend Tiffany and I were grilling some filet mignon and zucchini but we did not have any sauce. . . . So we started throwing the herbs Tiff had in her fridge into the blender and before we knew it we had an amazing chimichurri. We hope you enjoy it as much as we do! If you happen to have a Meyer lemon, use its juice for a really special flavor.

½ cup flat-leaf parsley leaves
¾ cup fresh cilantro leaves
⅓ cup fresh mint leaves
1 shallot, peeled
1 garlic clove, peeled
¼ jalapeño chile pepper, seeded
½ cup extra-virgin olive oil

1 tablespoon fresh lemon juice
½ teaspoon Sriracha sauce (Thai chili sauce)
½ teaspoon fine sea salt
½ teaspoon red pepper flakes
⅛ teaspoon cayenne pepper

Combine all the ingredients in a blender and blend for 30 seconds. Scrape the sides with a rubber spatula and blend again for 30 seconds, until the ingredients are well combined.

Nutrition facts per 2-tablespoon serving: 80 calories, 0 grams protein, 1 gram carbohydrates, 7 grams fat

Viva Italia Dressing

MAKES 2½ CUPS

To make a flavorful marinade for chicken or shrimp, double the herbs, add another clove or two of garlic, and process in a blender.

1¼ cups extra-virgin olive oil

⅓ cup red wine vinegar

3 garlic cloves, minced

2 tablespoons grated Parmesan cheese

¼ teaspoon black peppercorns

½ teaspoon fine sea salt

¼ teaspoon dried basil

¼ teaspoon dried oregano

¼ teaspoon dried rosemary

¼ teaspoon ground black pepper

Pinch of red pepper flakes

Combine all the ingredients in a blender and blend until smooth.

Nutrition facts per tablespoon: 100 calories, 0 grams protein, 0 grams carbohydrates, 11 grams fat (mostly good fats!)

Minted Greek Chicken

SERVES 6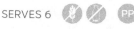

Mint's not just for mojitos and dessert garnishes anymore. It brightens up the flavor and adds a touch of summer to savory dishes too. If you are using wooden skewers, make sure you soak them for at least 30 minutes so they do not burn on the grill.

1½ pounds boneless, skinless chicken breasts, cut into 1-inch cubes

2 tablespoons extra-virgin olive oil

3 garlic cloves, crushed with the side of a knife

1 teaspoon dried mint

1 teaspoon dried oregano

1 teaspoon fine sea salt

1 teaspoon ground black pepper

2 tablespoons fresh lemon juice

1 bunch fresh mint

1 red onion, cut into 1-inch pieces

Combine the chicken, 1 tablespoon of the oil, the garlic, dried mint, oregano, salt, and pepper in a medium bowl. Toss well to coat, cover, and marinate in the refrigerator for at least 30 minutes and up to 24 hours.

Preheat a grill to medium-high. Whisk together the remaining 1 tablespoon oil and the lemon juice in a small bowl.

Pull the large mint leaves off the stems. Thread the chicken and onion onto twelve 8-inch skewers, threading a mint leaf in between the chicken and onion. Sprinkle with the salt and pepper.

Grill the kebabs, turning and basting with the lemon-oil mixture, until the chicken is cooked through, 9 to 10 minutes.

Nutrition facts per serving: 160 calories, 27 grams protein, 3 grams carbohydrates, 5 grams fat

PFC Hint: Serve over rice.

Ruby Red Yakitori Kebabs

SERVES 10

Nothing says summer like grilling, and nothing say yummy like my yakitori kebabs! Grilling is such a healthy alternative to pan-frying and other methods that often use extra fat to boost the flavors. The smokiness from the grill and all that Asian influence really pack a punch. Just remember you do not want to burn your skewers, so if you are using wooden ones, make sure to soak them for at least 30 minutes. This makes a lot, but leftovers make a great lunch for later in the week.

¾ cup low-sodium soy sauce

½ cup mirin or apple juice

¼ cup organic ketchup

2 tablespoons rice vinegar

2 garlic cloves, minced

1 teaspoon minced fresh ginger

1 teaspoon toasted sesame oil

2 pounds boneless, skinless chicken breasts or extra-firm tofu, cubed

1 yellow bell pepper, cut into 1-inch squares

1 orange bell pepper, cut into 1-inch squares

1 red onion, cut into 1-inch squares

Whisk together the soy sauce, mirin or apple juice, ketchup, vinegar, garlic, ginger, and sesame oil in a medium bowl. Place the chicken or tofu cubes in a large resealable plastic bag and pour in three-fourths of the marinade. Press most of the air out of the bag and seal tightly. In a separate bag, combine the peppers and onion and the remaining marinade. Press out the air and seal tightly. Refrigerate both the chicken and the peppers for 30 minutes to 2 hours, turning the bags occasionally to make sure everything marinates evenly.

Preheat the grill to medium-high. Thread the chicken, peppers, and onion alternately onto skewers. Discard the chicken marinade but reserve the vegetable marinade.

Lightly coat the kebabs with cooking spray. Turn the grill to medium and grill the kebabs over direct heat for 5 minutes. Turn, baste with the remaining marinade, and grill 5 minutes on the second side.

Nutrition facts per serving: 168 calories, 23 grams protein, 11 grams carbohydrates, 2 grams fat

PFC Hint: Serve the kebabs over quinoa or brown rice with a cucumber salad.

Grilled Halibut with Tomato Coulis

SERVES 4

Fish is one of my go-to proteins because it's so low in saturated fat. Some people are intimidated by fish, yet it is one of the quickest and easiest proteins to cook. So don't be scared—fish is your friend in the kitchen!

TOMATO COULIS

2 beefsteak tomatoes

¼ cup red wine vinegar

1 teaspoon minced garlic

1 teaspoon fine sea salt

½ teaspoon ground black pepper

1 red onion, chopped

¼ cup extra-virgin olive oil

HALIBUT

4 halibut fillets (4 ounces each)

Olive oil, for brushing

Sea salt and cracked black pepper

1 bunch fresh thyme

Juice of 1 lemon

To make the tomato coulis: Bring a pot of water to a boil. Fill a bowl with ice and water. Cut a shallow "X" at the bottom of each tomato. Add the tomatoes to the boiling water and blanch for 1 minute. Transfer to the ice water to cool, then peel. Halve the tomatoes through the equator, then squeeze out the juice and seeds. Finely dice the tomato flesh and place in a medium bowl. Stir in the vinegar and garlic and set aside for 30 minutes. Transfer the tomato mixture to a food processor, add the salt and pepper, and pulse to combine. Add the onion and then, with the machine running, slowly drizzle in the oil.

To prepare the halibut: Coat a fish grill basket with cooking spray and preheat your grill to medium-high. Brush the halibut fillets with oil and season lightly with salt and cracked pepper.

Place the bunch of thyme in the fish grill basket and place over the fire. Once the thyme starts smoking, place the fillets in the basket and place on the grill. Close the lid and grill for 6 minutes. Lift the lid and rotate the fish fillets 90 degrees to create crisscross grill marks and close the lid again. Grill the fish until it flakes easily, about 6 minutes. Serve the fish with tomato coulis and garnish with grilled thyme.

Nutrition facts per serving: 273 calories, 24 grams protein, 3 grams carbohydrates, 18 grams fat (all good fats!)

PFC Hint: Serve over rice or add a dessert.

Zesty Citrus Halibut on Asian Slaw

SERVES 5

I can't tell you how many times I have made this dish for my friends to rave reviews. The halibut is mild in flavor, so it is a great option for those who don't like "fishy" fish. Try to avoid Atlantic halibut because it is high in mercury—Alaskan halibut is the safest choice.

Grated zest and juice of 1 lime

Grated zest and juice of 1 orange

1 tablespoon coconut oil, melted

Fine sea salt and ground black pepper

1 pound halibut fillet

½ head Napa cabbage, shredded

Cilantro Chili Lime Dressing (page 227)

Stir together the lime zest, orange zest, coconut oil, and a pinch of sea salt and pepper. Coat the halibut with the mixture and marinate in the refrigerator for 20 minutes.

Place the cabbage in a bowl and drizzle with the dressing. Toss lightly. Set the slaw aside.

Heat a large skillet over medium-high heat. Add the fish and cook for 5 minutes. Flip the fillet and cook until the fish flakes easily, about 5 minutes. Cut into 5 portions and serve each on a bed of the slaw.

Nutrition facts per serving: 275 calories, 21 grams protein, 5 grams carbohydrates, 18 grams fat (all good fats!)

PFC Hint: Serve over rice.

Chef Cece's Bouillabaisse

SERVES 8

While I was attending Westlake Culinary Institute, this delicious, real-food soup was one of my favorite things we made, so I had to include it in this book even though it's not my recipe. It was created by my culinary instructor, chef Cecilia de Castro, who worked as Wolfgang Puck's assistant for over 20 years. Chef Cece's professional chef program has become so popular that she recently opened her own culinary school, the Academy of Culinary Education, where students get the opportunity to cook with Wolfgang and Sherry Yard for the Academy Awards every year. You can be sure that this bouillabaisse is beyond flavorful. Serve with fresh sourdough baguette.

¼ cup extra-virgin olive oil

½ medium onion, chopped

1 leek, white part only, chopped

2 garlic cloves, chopped

2 large tomatoes, seeded and chopped

1 cup fish stock, homemade or store-bought

2 sprigs thyme

¼ teaspoon saffron threads

Splash of Pernod

½ pound shell-on large shrimp

½ pound skinless sea bass fillets, cut into 3 x 1-inch strips

1 pound skinless sole fillets, cut into 3 x 1-inch strips

¼ pound crabmeat

Sea salt and ground black pepper

Heat the oil in a large pot over medium heat. Add the onion and leek and cook until softened, about 5 minutes. Add the garlic and cook for 2 minutes. Add the tomatoes and cook for 5 minutes. Stir in the stock, thyme, saffron, and Pernod and bring to a simmer. Add the shrimp, cover, and cook for 2 minutes. Add the fish and cook for 1 minute. Stir in the crab and season with sea salt and pepper to taste.

Nutrition facts per 1½-cup serving: 225 calories, 30 grams protein, 2 grams carbohydrates, 10 grams fat (all good fats!)

PFC Hint: Have with a medium size piece of crusty bread.

Mongolian Beef

SERVES 4

Not to toot my own horn, but I think this healthier alternative to what you get at most Chinese restaurants tastes loads better than your typical take-out! Making the sauce and cutting the veggies can be done hours ahead of time, which makes putting this meal together a snap.

¼ cup low-sodium soy sauce

1 tablespoon hoisin sauce

1 tablespoon rice vinegar

1 tablespoon cornstarch

1 tablespoon sambal (chili-garlic paste)

1 teaspoon coconut palm sugar or ½ teaspoon stevia

8 ounces rice noodles

2 teaspoons coconut oil

2 tablespoons minced garlic

2 tablespoons minced fresh ginger

1 pound grass fed sirloin steak, thinly sliced across the grain

16 scallions, cut into 2-inch pieces

2 carrots, diced

1 cup fresh bean sprouts

Combine the soy sauce, hoisin, vinegar, sambal, and sugar in a small bowl, stirring until smooth.

Bring a medium pot of water to a boil. Add the rice noodles and cook according to package directions. Drain and set aside.

Melt the coconut oil in a large nonstick skillet over medium-high heat. Add the garlic, ginger, and beef and cook until beef is browned, about 5 minutes. Add the veggies and cook for 30 seconds. Add the soy sauce mixture and cook, stirring constantly, until thickened, about 1 minute.

Remove from the heat, add the cooked noodles and bean sprouts, and toss to combine. Serve immediately.

Nutrition facts per serving: 210 calories, 21 grams protein, 19 grams carbohydrates, 5 grams fat

PFC Hint: Add rice or rice noodles.

Smoky Beef Stew

SERVES 10

I once babysat for a toddler who insisted on beef stew for lunch. I was panicked because his mom had outlined all of the lunch options (frozen nuggets, frozen burgers), none of which was beef stew. When his mom finally arrived home it was pointed out that there was a bountiful amount of canned beef stew in the cupboard. Yuck—I'd never heard of beef stew in a can. Beef stew is meant to be homemade and savored! This recipe is fantastic, and you will especially love the leftovers the next day. Serve with Chipotle Cheddar Cornbread (opposite).

2 pounds grass fed beef tenderloin or top sirloin, cut into ½-inch cubes

2 tablespoons olive oil

8 garlic cloves, minced

½ teaspoon fine sea salt

½ teaspoon ground black pepper

¼ teaspoon cayenne pepper

¼ teaspoon red pepper flakes

½ cup whole wheat flour

1 teaspoon fresh thyme leaves

1 large onion, chopped

1 can (14.5 ounces) diced fire-roasted tomatoes

1 can (15 ounces) tomato sauce

1 cup beef stock

3 russet (baking) potatoes (about 1½ pounds), peeled and cubed

4 carrots, sliced

2 teaspoons diced canned chipotles with 2 teaspoons of the adobo sauce

1½ cups frozen peas

1 cup frozen green beans

Combine the meat, 1 tablespoon of the oil, 2 of the chopped garlic cloves, the sea salt, black pepper, cayenne, and red pepper flakes in a medium bowl. Cover with plastic wrap and marinate for 1 to 2 hours in the fridge.

Remove the meat from the marinade. Dredge the beef in the flour and shake off the excess.

Heat a large pot or Dutch oven over medium-high heat. Add the remaining 1 tablespoon oil, the thyme, and meat. Cook the meat, turning, until browned on all sides, 10 to 15 minutes.

Add the onion and remaining garlic and cook until the onion has softened, about 5 minutes. Stir in the tomatoes, tomato sauce, stock, potatoes, carrots, and chipotles with adobo sauce. Bring to a boil then reduce to a simmer and cook for 40 minutes.

Add the peas and green beans and simmer for 5 minutes.

Nutrition facts per 1½-cup serving: 270 calories, 23 grams protein, 35 grams carbohydrates, 6 grams fat

Chipotle Cheddar Cornbread

MAKES 12 MUFFINS

These muffins are the perfect complement to any chili or stew. The chipotle in adobo factor provides a hit of heat, and there is a hint of sweetness from the coconut milk and white corn. If you like your corn muffins less sweet, replace the coconut milk with dairy milk.

1 cup whole wheat flour

1 cup yellow cornmeal

4 teaspoons baking powder

1 tablespoon Zsweet

¾ teaspoon fine sea salt

1½ cups coconut milk

2 tablespoons coconut oil, melted

1 large egg

½ cup frozen baby white corn kernels, thawed

¼ cup grated Cheddar cheese

2 teaspoons minced canned chipotles with 2 teaspoons of the adobo sauce

Preheat the oven to 425°F. Coat a 12-cup muffin pan with cooking spray.

Combine the flour, cornmeal, baking powder, Zsweet, and salt in a large bowl. Add the coconut milk, coconut oil, and egg and stir until combined, about 1 minute. Stir in the corn, cheese, and chipotles (and adobo sauce).

Scoop about ¼ cup batter into each muffin cup. Bake until a wooden pick inserted in a muffin comes out clean, 10 to 12 minutes. Cool the muffins in the pan for 5 minutes, then turn out onto a rack to cool completely.

Nutrition facts per muffin: 180 calories, 4 grams protein, 18 grams carbohydrates, 10 grams fat

PFC Hint: Pair with Smoky Beef Stew.

Christine's Pesto

MAKES ABOUT ½ CUP

2 cups tightly packed fresh basil leaves

½ cup grated Parmesan cheese

¼ cup pine nuts

¼ teaspoon cayenne pepper

1 garlic clove, crushed with the side of a knife

¼ cup extra-virgin olive oil

Sea salt and ground black pepper

Combine the basil, cheese, pine nuts, cayenne, and garlic in a food processor or blender. With the machine running, slowly pour in the oil. Blend until mixture looks bright green and thick, about 45 seconds. Season with salt and pepper to taste.

Nutrition facts per tablespoon: 71 calories, 1 gram protein, 1 gram carbohydrates, 7 grams fat (mostly good fats!)

Citrus-Soaked Pork Tacos

SERVES 8

I love Mexican food. Love it! Unfortunately, much of what is served in Mexican restaurants contains way too much saturated fat. My recipe replaces fat with flavor from all kinds of spices, herbs, and veggies. Achiote (also called annatto) is a seed that can be found in the Latin food aisle of most grocery stores or in any Latin market. One last bit of food for thought, on the subject of tortillas: Guerrero brand makes tortillas from real ingredients, so I always seek them out when I can.

MARINADE

½ teaspoon cumin seeds

½ teaspoon black peppercorns

2 tablespoons achiote (annatto seeds)

6 garlic cloves

1½ teaspoons coarse sea salt

¼ teaspoon ground cinnamon

1½ teaspoons dried oregano

⅓ cup fresh orange juice

¼ cup distilled white vinegar

TACOS

1 pound pork tenderloin

2 teaspoons olive oil

Sea salt and ground black pepper

1½ cups thinly sliced yellow onion

2 small jalapeño chile peppers, seeded and chopped

1 cup chicken stock

½ cup chopped fresh cilantro

¼ cup fresh lime juice

8 corn tortillas (6-inch)

2 cups shredded lettuce

1 cup fresh tomato salsa

To make the marinade: Toast the cumin and peppercorns in a dry skillet over medium heat until fragrant, 1 to 2 minutes. Finely grind the toasted spices and achiote using a mortar and pestle or a spice grinder. Mince the garlic and mash to a paste with the salt using the back of a spoon or a knife. Transfer the garlic paste to a shallow 13 x 9 x 2-inch baking dish. Stir in the spice mixture, the cinnamon, oregano, orange juice, vinegar, and ½ cup water.

To make the taco mixture: Add the pork to the marinade and rub the marinade all over the meat. Cover and marinate in the refrigerator for at least 2 hours.

Heat a large skillet over medium-high heat. Remove the pork from the marinade and pat dry with paper towels. Add the oil to the pan. Sprinkle the pork with salt and pepper, add to the pan and cook until the pork is browned on all sides, about 4 minutes. Transfer the pork to a cutting board to rest.

Add the onion and jalapeños to the pan and cook until the onion is tender, about 5 minutes.

Meanwhile, cut the pork into thin strips. Add the chicken stock to the skillet, reduce the heat and simmer for 1 minute. Return the pork strips to the pan. Stir in the cilantro and lime juice, cook for 1 minute, and remove from the heat.

Warm the tortillas directly over a stovetop burner or according to package directions. To serve, spoon ½ cup of pork mixture into each tortilla. Garnish with shredded lettuce and salsa.

Nutrition facts per taco: 212 calories, 19 grams protein, 18 grams carbohydrates, 7 grams fat

PFC Hint: Add some black beans.

Herb-Crusted Rack of Lamb with Açaí Sauce

SERVES 8

Lamb, like other strong-flavored meats, pairs well with a berry-based sauce because the acidity of the berry balances the richness of the meat. Though açaí berry juice is available at most supermarkets, if you cannot find it, use pomegranate juice (the nutrition facts will remain the same).

Two 8-rib racks of lamb (1½ pounds each)

2 tablespoons finely chopped fresh oregano

2 tablespoons finely chopped fresh parsley

2 tablespoons finely chopped fresh thyme

2 teaspoons Dijon mustard

2 large garlic cloves, minced

1 tablespoon plus 2 teaspoons sherry vinegar

1 teaspoon fine sea salt

1 teaspoon ground black pepper

¼ cup Port wine

2 shallots, finely chopped

½ cup chicken stock

1 cup açaí berry juice

1 teaspoon unsalted butter (preferably organic)

Preheat the oven to 400°F. Slice the fat from the top (convex) side of the bones by keeping the knife blade flush against the bone and following the contour of the bone. Trim the fat from between the ribs and scrape the bones clean for an elegant presentation.

Mix together the oregano, parsley, thyme, mustard, garlic, and 1 tablespoon of the vinegar in a bowl. Sprinkle the lamb with ½ teaspoon each of the salt and pepper.

Heat a large ovenproof skillet over medium heat. Coat the pan with cooking spray. Add the lamb meaty side down and cook until lightly browned, about 2 minutes. Transfer the racks to a cutting board and cover the meat on both sides with the herb mixture, patting to adhere. Return the racks to the pan and transfer the skillet to the oven. Roast until a thermometer inserted into the center of the lamb registers 138°F, 10 to 15 minutes.

Transfer the racks to a plate and cover with foil. Let the meat rest for 10 minutes, then cut into individual chops.

Meanwhile, return the skillet to medium heat (remember the handle will be hot!). Add the remaining 2 teaspoons vinegar, the Port, and shallots. Bring to a boil and cook until reduced by half, 5 to 7 minutes. Stir in the stock and cook for 5 to 7 minutes to reduce. Add the açaí juice and the remaining ½ teaspoon each salt and pepper and cook for 2 minutes. Add the butter and stir until melted. Serve the sauce with the lamb.

Nutrition facts per 2-rib serving: 220 calories, 22 grams protein, 7 grams carbohydrates, 11 grams fat

PFC Hint: Add a few roasted potatoes.

Grilled Margarita Pizzas

SERVES 8

The amount of pizza we Americans consume annually would cover the equivalent of 100 football fields—about 100 acres! Why? Because it tastes so darn good. Sadly, most commercial pizzas contain a plethora of unpronounceable ingredients, large amounts of salt, unhealthy trans fats, and food coloring. Let's get real, people! Make your own pizza! If you use real ingredients, you are sure to look and feel phenomenal. Bonus: The fresh basil on this pizza can help reduce coughs and constipation. You can also make this on a ridged grill pan.

1 pound refrigerated or thawed
    frozen whole wheat pizza dough

2 cups bottled pizza sauce (see Note)

12 small mozzarella balls
    (bocconcini), halved

24 cherry tomatoes, halved

2 cups basil leaves, finely shredded

Place the dough on a floured work surface and divide into 8 portions. Let the dough rest for 20 minutes. Set the bocconcini on paper towels to drain (this will prevent your pizza from getting soggy in the middle).

Preheat a grill to high.

Flatten each ball of dough into a large round. Generously coat on both sides with olive oil cooking spray. Gently lift the rounds and set on the grill over direct heat. Cover the grill and cook, without turning, until the dough has puffed up and grill marks appear on the bottom, about 3 minutes.

Transfer the grilled pizza rounds to a baking sheet with the grilled side up. Place 3 tablespoons pizza sauce, 6 halved mozzarella balls, and 6 cherry tomato halves on each pizza.

Carefully transfer the topped pizzas to the grill, cover, and grill, rotating once for even cooking, until the bottom is browned and crisp. Serve topped with fresh basil.

Note: Read labels carefully to find a pizza sauce with all real ingredients.

Nutrition facts per pizza: 240 calories, 12 grams protein, 30 grams carbohydrates, 9 grams fat

Easy Lobster Pasta

SERVES 6

Lobster is expensive, so this is a great way to make a little bit of lobster go a long way. You will want the pasta to finish cooking right around the time the lobster mixture finishes, so if you use a different type of pasta, plan ahead. BTW, this is really yummolicious served with grilled endive or escarole.

1 tablespoon plus 1 teaspoon fine sea salt

1 pound capellini or other strand pasta

1 whole 2-pound lobster, steamed or boiled (about 16 minutes)

1 tablespoon unsalted butter (preferably organic)

1 shallot, thinly sliced, or ¼ white or red onion

3 garlic cloves, minced or pressed

½ teaspoon red pepper flakes

1 tablespoon extra-virgin olive oil

1 handful flat-leaf parsley, chopped

Zest and juice of 1 lemon (optional)

Bring a large pot of water to a boil and add 1 tablespoon of the salt. Add the capellini and cook for 1 to 2 minutes, checking the texture after 1 minute. If it's still too firm, continue cooking, but check every 30 seconds until just al dente (the texture of the pasta can make or break this dish).

While the pasta water is coming to a boil, remove the lobster meat from its shell and chop into bite-size pieces. Melt the butter in a large skillet over medium heat. Add the shallot, garlic, red pepper flakes and remaining 1 teaspoon salt. Cook until the garlic is golden brown, about 2 minutes. Add the lobster meat and cook for 1 minute. Turn off the heat and stir in the oil.

Drain the pasta and using tongs, toss with the parsley with the warm lobster mixture. Sprinkle with the lemon zest and juice if desired. Serve immediately.

Nutrition facts per serving: 410 calories, 25 grams protein, 61 grams carbohydrates, 7 grams fat

Cilantro-Lime Shrimp with Spicy Rice Noodles

SERVES 4

Rice noodles are most commonly used in Asian cuisine. The principle ingredients are rice and water. You can find them in the Asian foods aisle of your grocery store. If you are meal planning for the week, buy 1 pound of shrimp and grill them all at once, setting aside about ¼ pound to use in a salad or pasta dish later in the week.

8 ounces rice noodles

¼ cup coconut oil, melted

3 tablespoons low-sodium soy sauce

3 tablespoons tamari

1 teaspoon raw organic honey

1 teaspoon Sriracha sauce (Thai chili sauce)

¼ teaspoon wasabi paste

2 large shallots, thinly sliced and separated into rings

6 garlic cloves, coarsely chopped

Grated zest and juice of 2 limes, plus lime wedges for serving

¾ pound large shrimp, peeled and deveined

Sea salt and ground black pepper

2 scallions, finely chopped

½ cup chopped fresh cilantro

¼ teaspoon red pepper flakes

Bring a large pot of water to a boil. Add the noodles and cook, stirring, until tender, about 2 minutes. Drain.

Combine 2 tablespoons of the coconut oil, the soy sauce, tamari, honey, Sriracha, and wasabi paste in a medium bowl. Add the noodles and toss. Set aside.

Heat 1 tablespoon of coconut oil in a large skillet over medium heat. Add the shallots and cook, stirring, until golden brown and crisp, about 3 minutes. Using a slotted spoon, transfer the shallots to paper towels to drain. Add the garlic to the skillet and cook over low heat until just golden and crisp, about 2 minutes. Transfer the garlic to paper towels to drain.

Preheat a grill or a ridged grill pan over high heat. Combine the lime zest and juice and the remaining 1 tablespoon oil in a medium bowl. Stir in the shrimp and season with salt and pepper. Grill the shrimp, turning once, until glazed and just opaque throughout, about 3 minutes.

Arrange the noodles on a large platter. Sprinkle with the scallions, cilantro, red pepper flakes, and the fried shallots and garlic. Arrange the shrimp on top and serve with lime wedges alongside.

Nutrition facts per serving: 480 calories, 28 grams protein, 54 grams carbohydrates, 16 grams fat (all good fats!)

Farmers' Market Veggie Pasta

SERVES 7

Pesto has such intense flavor that a little goes a long way. Fortunately, most of the prepared pesto sauces found in the refrigerator sections of the grocery store have the same ingredients as homemade pesto and are therefore still real food; just take a good look at the ingredient list to be sure. You'll see I also have you cooking the pasta in the same water you use to cook the asparagus—this will boost the flavor of the pasta and will conserve a little water as well.

1 pound asparagus, cut into 1-inch pieces

1 pound whole wheat penne pasta

2 tablespoons extra-virgin olive oil

8 ounces water-packed or thawed frozen artichoke hearts, quartered

1 red onion, thinly sliced into rounds

¼ cup vegetable stock or your favorite white wine

¼ cup Christine's Pesto (see page 238) or store-bought pesto

¾ cup shredded reduced-fat mozzarella cheese

Bring a large pot of salted water to a boil. Add the asparagus and boil for 1 minute. Remove the asparagus with a slotted spoon and run under cold water to stop the cooking.

Bring the same pot of water back to a boil and add the penne. Cook until al dente, according to package directions. Drain and set aside.

Heat an extra-large skillet over medium-high and add the oil. Add the asparagus, artichoke hearts and onion and cook until the onion begins to caramelize, 5 to 7 minutes. (If you don't have an extra-large skillet, do this in batches.) Add the stock or wine and cook for 1 to 2 minutes, scraping up all the browned bits from the pan. Stir in the pesto and cook gently until the pesto is evenly distributed. Add the pasta and toss with tongs until the vegetables and pasta are combined.

Divide among 7 bowls and sprinkle with the mozzarella.

Nutrition facts per serving: 370 calories, 18 grams protein, 53 grams carbohydrates, 10 grams fat

Roasted Vegetable Lasagna

SERVES 10

My best friend Lily, who has a severe gluten allergy, raves about my lasagna and finds it hard to believe there is no gluten—it tastes that authentic! To get even, thin slices on the veggies, I recommend using a mandoline—it saves a ton of time.

Olive oil, for greasing the dish

6 medium red potatoes, very thinly sliced

Christine's Pesto (page 238)

Sea salt

¾ pound eggplant (about 1 large), unpeeled, thinly sliced

2 medium golden zucchini, thinly sliced

1 large red or yellow onion, thinly sliced

1 jar (24 ounces) marinara sauce

12 ounces soft goat cheese

Preheat the oven to 375°F. Grease a 2-quart baking dish with olive oil.

Arrange half the potato slices in the dish. Season each potato with a small drop of the pesto. Top each potato with a slice of eggplant, zucchini, and onion. Using half the goat cheese, place a bit of cheese onto the top of each vegetable stack. Pour half of the marinara over everything. Make a second layer of potatoes, pesto, vegetables, and sauce. Lastly, drop mini dollops of the remaining 6 ounces of goat cheese over the top of the lasagna.

Cover the dish with foil and bake for 45 minutes. Remove the foil and bake until the lasagna is bubbling and the top has browned, about 10 minutes.

Nutrition facts per serving: 297 calories, 12 grams protein, 35 grams carbohydrates, 13 grams fat

Lemonata Raspberry Bread Pudding

SERVES 12

The bread pudding can be served warm or cold and it's especially good with vanilla ice cream on top. Decorate each serving with a mint sprig and fresh raspberries for special occasions.

3¼ cups 1% or 2% milk

3 large eggs (preferably cage free)

4 egg whites (preferably from cage free eggs)

1 cup coconut palm sugar

¼ cup fresh lemon juice (about 2 lemons)

Grated zest of 2 lemons

1 vanilla bean, split

1 pound stale whole wheat bread, cut into cubes

2 cups raspberries, fresh or frozen

Fresh mint, for garnish

Preheat the oven to 400°F. Coat a 9 x 13-inch baking dish with cooking spray.

Whisk together 3 cups of the milk, the whole eggs, egg whites, sugar, lemon zest, and lemon juice in a large bowl.

Warm the remaining ¼ cup milk in a small saucepan over low heat until lukewarm, scrape the seeds from the vanilla bean into the warming milk and gently stir to separate. Remove from the heat and stir into the egg and lemon mixture.

Place the bread cubes in the baking dish. Pour the egg mixture over the bread and set aside for 20 minutes to allow the bread to absorb the liquid. Add the raspberries to the bread mixture and toss gently.

Cover the baking dish with foil and bake for 20 minutes. Uncover and bake until slightly puffed and golden, 10 to 15 minutes.

Nutrition facts per serving: 216 calories, 11 grams protein, 36 grams carbohydrates, 4 grams fat

PFC Hint: Indulge after a PP meal or omit the carb from a PC meal.

Raspberry-Kissed Brownies

MAKES 12 BROWNIES

Gluten free flour is a combination of garbanzo bean flour, potato starch, tapioca flour, sorghum flour, and fava bean flour, making it wheat free. If you don't want to use gluten free flour, simply swap in whole wheat flour and omit the xanthan. The gluten free flour and xanthan gum can be found in most grocery stores in the baking aisle.

½ cup gluten free flour

¼ teaspoon xanthan gum

¼ teaspoon baking powder

¼ teaspoon fine sea salt

1 cup coconut palm sugar

⅔ cup pureed canned organic sweet potatoes

1 large egg

1 egg white

1½ teaspoons pure vanilla extract

¼ teaspoon instant espresso powder

3 tablespoons unsalted butter (preferably organic)

1 tablespoon coconut oil, melted

⅔ cup unsweetened cocoa powder

⅔ cup fresh raspberries

Preheat the oven to 350°F. Coat an 8-inch square baking pan with cooking spray.

Whisk together the flour, xanthan gum, baking powder, and salt in a small bowl.

Stir together the sugar and sweet potatoes in a medium bowl until well combined. Beat in the whole egg and egg white. Mix together the vanilla and espresso powder in a small bowl until the powder is dissolved.

Melt the butter in a medium saucepan over low heat. Remove from the heat and stir in the coconut oil. Slowly stir in the cocoa powder, stirring with a fork until the chocolate mixture resembles a thick smooth sauce. Stir in the espresso-vanilla mixture.

Combine the flour mixture with the sweet potato mixture until no trace of the flour remains. Stir in the chocolate mixture and mix until the batter is dark brown. Carefully fold in the raspberries. Spoon the batter into the baking pan and smooth the top with a spatula coated with cooking spray. Bake until a wooden pick inserted in the center of the brownies comes out clean, 25 to 30 minutes. Cool and cut into 12 brownies.

Nutrition facts per brownie: 139 calories, 3 grams protein, 25 grams carbohydrates, 5 grams fat

PFC Hint: Indulge after a PP meal or omit the carb from a PC meal.

Cocoberry Cupcakes

MAKES 18 CUPCAKES

A few notes about these cupcakes: There is refined sugar in the frosting, one of the few times it is used in this book, but it is necessary in this case to achieve a smooth frosting. Second, coconut palm sugar can usually be found at places like Whole Foods and at Asian markets. This recipe can be made 1 day ahead. Store in the refrigerator in airtight containers. Bring to room temperature before serving.

CUPCAKES

2 cans (13 to 14 ounces each) light coconut milk

2 cups whole wheat flour

2¼ teaspoons baking powder

½ teaspoon fine sea salt

1 stick (4 ounces) unsalted butter (preferably organic), at room temperature

¼ cup coconut oil, melted

¾ cup coconut palm sugar

½ cup Zsweet

3 large eggs (preferably cage free)

Seeds scraped from 1 vanilla bean or 1 teaspoon pure vanilla extract

FROSTING AND GARNISH

1 stick (4 ounces) unsalted butter (preferably organic), at room temperature

1¼ cups organic confectioners' sugar

Seeds scraped from 1 vanilla bean or 1 teaspoon pure vanilla extract

⅛ teaspoon fine sea salt

1 pint blueberries

1 pint raspberries

¾ cup unsweetened flaked coconut, lightly toasted, for garnish

To make the cupcakes: Bring the coconut milk to a boil in large deep saucepan over medium-high heat (use a deep pan because it will boil up in the pan). Reduce the heat to medium-low and boil until reduced to 1½ cups, 25 to 30 minutes, stirring occasionally. Remove from the heat and cool completely. Transfer to a small bowl. Cover and refrigerate (the coconut milk will settle slightly as it cools). This can be done up to 2 days ahead of time; cover and keep chilled in the refrigerator. If the reduced coconut milk is lumpy when you're ready to use it, process in a food processor for about 20 seconds to smooth it out.

Position a rack in the center of the oven and preheat to 350°F. Line 18 muffin cups with paper liners.

Whisk together the flour, baking powder, and salt in a medium bowl. Using an electric mixer, beat the butter and coconut oil in a large bowl until smooth. Add the coconut sugar and Zsweet and beat on medium-high speed until well blended, about 2 minutes. Add 2 of the eggs, 1 at a time, beating well after each addition and occasionally scraping down the sides of the bowl. Beat in the seeds from the vanilla bean or the extract and the remaining egg. Add half of the flour mixture and mix on low speed just until blended. Add 1 cup of the reduced coconut milk and mix just until blended. (Reserve the remaining reduced coconut milk to use in the frosting.) Add the remaining flour mixture and mix on low speed just until blended.

Divide the batter among the muffin cups. Bake until the tops spring back when gently touched and a wooden pick inserted in the center comes out clean, about 20 minutes. Cool the cupcakes in the pans on a rack for 10 minutes. Then transfer the cupcakes to the rack to cool completely.

To make the frosting: Using an electric mixer, beat the butter in a large bowl until smooth. Add the confectioners' sugar, 2 tablespoons of the reserved reduced coconut milk, the seeds from the vanilla bean or extract, and salt. Beat on medium-low speed until blended, scraping down the sides of the bowl. Increase the speed to medium-high and beat until light and fluffy.

Using a pastry bag fitted with a large star tip, pipe frosting onto the cooled cupcakes. Alternatively, use a small offset spatula to swirl the frosting over the top of the cupcakes. Decorate each cupcake with a few berries and sprinkle with coconut.

Nutrition facts per cupcake: 190 calories, 3 grams protein, 23 grams carbohydrate, 11 grams fat

PFC Hint: Indulge after a PP meal or omit the carb from a PC meal.

White Peach and Bing Cherry Cobbler

SERVES 9

Consider this dessert the carbohydrate portion of a healthful summer "pc combo" meal. Peach cobbler is a fantastic ending to a meal of grilled fish or chicken. If you can't find white peaches, use yellow; it will be just as delicious.

4 white peaches, peeled and cubed

2 cups Bing cherries, pitted

½ teaspoon grated lemon zest

Juice of 1 lemon

¼ cup plus ⅓ cup coconut palm sugar or Zsweet

½ teaspoon ground cinnamon

2 tablespoons plus 1¼ cups whole wheat flour

½ teaspoon baking powder

¼ teaspoon fine sea salt

3 tablespoons cold unsalted butter (preferably organic), cut into small pieces

½ cup low-fat buttermilk

1 tablespoon turbinado sugar (also called Raw Sugar)

Preheat the oven to 400°F. Coat an 8 x 8-inch square baking pan with butter-flavored cooking spray.

Combine the peaches, cherries, lemon zest, lemon juice, ¼ cup of the sugar, 2 tablespoons of the whole wheat flour, and the cinnamon in a bowl. Toss to coat the fruit evenly. Pour into the baking dish and bake for 15 minutes.

Meanwhile, combine the remaining 1¼ cups flour, the remaining ⅓ cup sugar, baking powder, and salt in a medium bowl. Cut in the chilled butter with a pastry blender or by cross-cutting it with 2 knives. Add the buttermilk and ½ cup water, stirring to make a slightly moist batter.

Remove the fruit from the oven and using a large spoon, arrange 8 dollops of the topping evenly over the fruit, leaving a 1-inch border around the baking dish. Sprinkle the dough with the turbinado sugar.

Return to the oven and bake until the top is golden brown and the fruit filling is bubbling, 25 minutes.

Nutrition facts per serving: 146 calories, 4 grams protein, 25 grams carbohydrates, 5 grams fat

PFC Hint: Indulge after a PP meal or omit the carb from a PC meal.

Persimmon Party Cookies

MAKES 60 MINIATURE COOKIES

We had a huge persimmon tree on our ranch and when they were ripe my grand-mother would simply dig a spoon into one and enjoy it as if it were a cup of pud-ding. She also used them to make smoothies. However I liked them best in her famous persimmon cookies. I've altered her original recipe here to offer a lighter, lower-sugar version and I must admit they taste just as delicious as Nonna's.

2 cups persimmon pulp (from about 4 medium persimmons)

1 cup coconut palm sugar

1 cup Zsweet

4 tablespoons (½ stick) unsalted butter (preferably organic), at room temperature

½ cup coconut oil, melted

2 large eggs (preferably cage free)

2 egg whites (preferably from cage free eggs)

3½ cups whole wheat flour

2 teaspoons baking powder

2 teaspoons ground cinnamon

1 teaspoon ground nutmeg

1¼ cups chopped walnuts

1 cup raisins

Preheat the oven to 375°F.

Combine the persimmon pulp, sugar, Zsweet, butter, and coconut oil in a blender and process until well blended but not frothy. Pour into a medium bowl. Slowly whisk in the eggs and egg whites.

Stir together the flour, baking powder, cinnamon, and nutmeg and baking powder in a separate medium bowl. Add to the persimmon mixture and mix well. Fold in the walnuts and raisins.

Drop the batter by the teaspoonful about 1 inch apart onto an ungreased baking sheet. Bake until the cookies are golden brown, about 15 minutes. The cookies should be a little soft so be careful to not overbake. Cool on the baking sheets for 10 minutes then transfer to a rack to cool completely.

Nutrition facts per 3-cookie serving: 140 calories, 3 grams protein, 17 grams carbohydrates, 7 grams fat

PFC Hint: Indulge after a PP meal or omit the carb from a PC meal.

Icy Watermelon Coconut Granita

SERVES 8

Here's the skinny on watermelon. . . . Webmd.com calls watermelon one of the best summer weight loss foods, and at 72 percent water, common sense would agree. But there is so much more to this lusciously sweet, crisp, and refreshing treat. It not only tastes fabulous (I've never met anyone who dislikes watermelon, have you?), but it is packed with disease-fighting antioxidants like vitamin C, and contains more lycopene than any other fresh fruit or vegetable. Simply speaking, that's more nutrition per calorie than most other fruits.

Watermelon's megadose of antioxidants neutralizes free radicals, substances in the body that promote premature aging and disease. A 2003 study in the Journal of Nutrition *showed that regular consumption of watermelon juice reduced the risks of high blood pressure, heart disease, and certain cancers.*

The natural sweetness found in watermelon can satisfy a nagging sweet tooth and help you resist factory-made sweets filled with trans fats, refined white sugar, and high fructose corn syrup. Watermelon is also high in potassium, which helps reduce water retention and bloating.

4 cups cubed, seeded watermelon

½ cup light coconut milk

1 tablespoon fresh lime juice

5 tablespoons maple syrup, honey, or Zsweet

Place the watermelon in a blender and puree. Add the coconut milk, lime juice, and sweetener and blend for 10 more seconds; do not blend longer or the mixture will turn foamy. Pour the mixture into an 8 x 8-inch metal baking dish. Freeze for 2 hours. Scrape with a fork to create crystals and return to the freezer. Continue to scrape and refreeze every 30 minutes for another 2 hours.

Nutrition facts per ½-cup serving: 70 calories, 0 grams protein, 18 grams carbohydrates, 1 gram fat

Variation: You can also freeze the mixture (made without the lime juice) in popsicle molds to make a great treat for kids—or watermelon lovers of any age.

PFC Hint: Indulge after a PP meal or omit the carb from a PC meal.

Tipsy Pear Sorbet

SERVES 7

Bartlett pears work especially well for this sorbet because they have a sweet yet subtle hint of tartness that pairs (no pun intended) nicely with the pinot grigio. If you cannot find Bartlett pears, experiment with a different variety. You can make this up to 1 week ahead.

1 lemon

½ cup Zsweet

1¼ pounds Bartlett pears, unpeeled, cored, and cut into cubes

¾ cup pinot grigio or other dry white wine

¼ teaspoon kosher salt

Mint leaves, for garnish

With a vegetable peeler, peel off thin strips of lemon zest to use as a garnish. Juice the lemon.

Combine 1 cup of water and the Zsweet in a medium saucepan and bring to a boil over medium-high heat. Add the pears and reduce the heat to a simmer. Cook, partially covered, until the pear cubes are very tender, 10 to 15 minutes. Remove from the heat and stir in the lemon juice, wine, and salt.

Press the pear mixture and cooking liquid through a fine mesh strainer or pass through a food milk into a bowl to remove the skins. Whisk to blend evenly.

Pour the puree into a 9 x 13-inch glass baking dish and freeze for 20 minutes. Pour into an ice cream maker and freeze according to the manufacturer's instructions until thickened, 25 to 30 minutes. For a firmer texture, transfer to an airtight container and freeze for another 8 hours before serving.

Serve garnished with a twist of lemon zest and fresh mint leaves.

Nutrition facts per ½-cup serving: 78 calories, 0 grams protein, 15 grams carbohydrates, 0 grams fat

PFC Hint: Indulge after a PP meal or omit the carb from a PC meal.

Santorini Lemon-Feta Dip

MAKES ABOUT 1½ CUPS

You could serve this dip to a junk food lover and they would indulge happily, never knowing that it is actually healthy!

1 can (15 ounces) cannellini beans

1 cup crumbled low-fat feta cheese

Grated zest and juice of 1 lemon

¼ cup extra-virgin olive oil

¼ cup minced flat-leaf parsley, plus more for garnish

¼ cup fresh oregano leaves, minced

2 garlic cloves

Fine sea salt and ground black pepper

Combine the beans, cheese, lemon zest, lemon juice, oil, parsley, oregano, and garlic in a food processor. Puree until smooth. Season with salt and pepper to taste.

Scoop the dip into a shallow bowl and garnish with parsley.

Nutrition facts per tablespoon: 70 calories, 3 grams protein, 4 grams carbohydrates, 5 grams fat

PFC Hint: Great to pair with whole wheat pita chips or cucumber slices.

Whole Wheat Pita Chips

MAKES 64 CHIPS

Store these in an airtight container for up to a week.

8 whole wheat pita breads, cut into wedges

1 tablespoons extra-virgin olive oil

1 teaspoon paprika

1 tablespoon dried oregano

Preheat the oven to 400°F.

Toss together the pita wedges with the oil, paprika, and oregano in a large bowl. Spread on a baking sheet and bake until golden brown, about 20 minutes.

Nutrition facts for a 5-chip serving: 120 calories, 4 grams protein, 24 grams carbohydrates, 1 gram fat

PFC Hint: Great with Santorini Lemon-Feta Dip.

Fire-Roasted Salsa Verde
with Skinny Chips

SERVES 8

These chips are naturally high in fiber, low in sodium, low in fat! And homemade fresh salsa is virtually sodium free and contains zero preservatives.

SALSA VERDE

7 fresh tomatillos, papery husks removed

1 fresh Anaheim chile pepper

6 garlic cloves, peeled but left whole

4 plum tomatoes

Fine sea salt and ground black pepper

1 bunch fresh cilantro, coarsely chopped

SKINNY CHIPS

10 corn tortillas (6-inch), cut into 8 wedges each

Fine sea salt and ground black pepper

To make the salsa verde: Preheat the oven to 400°F. Coat a baking sheet with cooking spray.

Arrange the tomatillos, chile, garlic, and tomatoes on the baking sheet and coat lightly with cooking spray. Season with salt and black pepper to taste.

Roast until the vegetables are soft and the skins of the tomatillos, chile, and tomatoes are beginning to take on color, about 15 minutes. If the chile begins to turn brown, remove it and continue roasting the tomatillos, tomatoes, and garlic. Remove the vegetables from the oven and turn the oven to broil. Return the vegetables (including the chile) to the oven and broil until lightly charred on one side. Important: Do not walk away from the oven while the vegetables are broiling because they will go from charred to burned in a matter of seconds. Set the vegetables aside to cool for 5 minutes. Leave the oven on, but reduce to 400°F.

Transfer the tomatillos, tomatoes, and garlic to a blender or food processor. Chop the roasted chile and add about 1 tablespoon to the blender. Blend for about 30 seconds. Taste, and if you want it spicier, keep blending in more chopped chile a tablespoon at a time until it's spicy enough for you. (Don't throw the entire chile into the blender or your salsa will be too fiery hot and bitter.) Mix in one handful of cilantro and salt and black pepper to taste.

To make the skinny chips: Coat a baking sheet with olive oil cooking spray. Spread the tortilla wedges evenly on the pan and coat lightly with cooking spray. Sprinkle with salt and pepper and bake until crispy, 10 to 15 minutes. Note: You do not need to turn the chips as they bake.

Cool the chips for 5 minutes and serve with the salsa.

Nutrition facts per serving (10 chips and ¼ cup salsa): 106 calories, 2 grams protein, 21 grams carbohydrates, 2 grams fat

PFC HInt: Serve as an appetizer with a lean protein dinner such as grilled fish or poultry.

Purple Passion Quesadillas

SERVES 4

Make these ahead of time and simply reheat them in your toaster oven for a smart, easy snack any time. I have found several brands of reduced-fat cheese that contain 100 percent real ingredients, so shop around and read labels; I'm positive you will find some at your local grocer. If you are still unsure of which brand to buy, www.labelwatch.com is a wonderful Web site that can be a great resource for finding 100 percent real food packaged goods.

4 slices (¼-inch thick) red onion

4 crosswise slices (¼-inch thick) eggplant

4 crosswise slices (¼-inch thick) golden zucchini

Fine sea salt and ground black pepper

8 corn tortillas (6-inch); Guerrero brand is 100 percent real/safe ingredients

½ cup grated reduced-fat Monterey Jack cheese

½ cup grated reduced-fat sharp Cheddar cheese

Fire Roasted Salsa Verde (see page 258) (optional)

¼ cup sour cream or Greek yogurt (optional)

Chopped fresh cilantro (optional)

4 lime wedges (optional)

Preheat the oven to 400°F. Coat a baking sheet with cooking spray.

Coat both sides of the vegetable slices with cooking spray. Sprinkle both sides with salt and pepper. Arrange on the baking sheet in a single layer and roast until tender and golden, 10 to 15 minutes. Remove from the oven and set aside.

Coat 4 of the tortillas with cooking spray and place them, oiled side down, on a baking sheet.

Combine the cheeses in a small bowl. Sprinkle ¼ cup cheese mixture over each of the tortillas on the baking sheet. Top each with 1 onion slice, 1 eggplant slice, and 1 zucchini slice. Top with the remaining tortillas. Coat the tops of the quesadillas with cooking spray.

Bake the quesadillas until the tortillas are slightly crisp and the cheese melts, about 10 minutes. Cut the quesadillas into quarters and garnish each serving with salsa, 1 tablespoon sour cream or Greek yogurt, and cilantro if desired. Serve with a lime wedge.

Nutrition facts per serving: 311 calories, 24 grams protein, 35 grams carbohydrates, 8 grams fat

Ole Guacamole

SERVES 4

Holy guacamole this dip is good! And the healthy fats in avocado make it guilt free too.

2 white corn tortillas (6-inch), cut into 8 wedges each

Fine sea salt and ground black pepper

2 teaspoons chopped fresh cilantro

2 teaspoons finely diced red onion

2 teaspoons seeded and minced jalapeño chile pepper

2 Hass avocados, cubed

1 lime, halved

Preheat the oven to 400°F. Coat a baking sheet with olive oil cooking spray. Spread the tortilla wedges evenly on the pan and coat lightly with cooking spray. Sprinkle with salt and pepper and bake until crispy, 10 to 15 minutes. Note: You do not need to turn the chips as they bake; that will only cause them to bend and look ugly (been there done that). Cool for 5 minutes.

Combine 1 teaspoon each of the cilantro, onion, and jalapeño with ½ teaspoon salt and ¼ teaspoon black pepper in a medium bowl and mash together with the back of a spoon. Add the avocados and gently mash them with a fork until they are somewhat smooth but still slightly chunky. Fold in the remaining 1 teaspoon each cilantro, onion, and jalapeño, and salt and pepper to taste. Squeeze in lime juice to taste. Serve with the warm chips.

Nutrition facts per serving (4 chips and ½ cup guacamole): 152 calories, 2 grams protein, 14 carbohydrates, 11 grams fat

PFC Hint: Great with Skinny Chips.

Heirloom Mac 'n' Cheese Muffins

MAKES ABOUT 36 MUFFINS

These muffins are a hit with everyone, 8 or 88! If you bake up a batch for a party, make sure you eat one before putting them out, because they will be gone in a flash! For really special occasions, I add a pound of diced cooked lobster meat instead of tomatoes.

1 pound whole wheat elbow macaroni

4 teaspoons olive oil

1 shallot, finely diced

2 garlic cloves, minced

1½ cups half-and-half

1½ cups 1% milk

3 tablespoons unsalted butter (preferably organic)

5 tablespoons whole wheat flour

1 pound reduced-fat sharp Cheddar cheese, grated

½ pound Gruyère cheese, grated

1 tablespoon coarse sea salt

½ teaspoon ground black pepper

3 large heirloom tomatoes, diced

¼ cup seasoned dried breadcrumbs

3 teaspoons minced fresh thyme leaves

Preheat the oven to 375°F. Coat three 12-cup muffin pans (disposable aluminum pans will work fine for this) with cooking spray.

In a large pot of boiling water, cook the pasta until al dente, according to package directions. Drain well.

Meanwhile, heat 1 teaspoon of the oil in a small skillet over medium heat. Add the shallot and garlic and cook until translucent, about 5 minutes. Set aside.

Combine the half-and-half and milk in a small saucepan and heat over medium heat; do not let boil. Keep warm.

Heat the butter and 2 teaspoons of the oil in a large pot over low heat. Whisk in the flour and cook, whisking frequently, until the mixture thickens and turns a very pale yellow, about 5 minutes. Add the sautéed shallot-garlic mixture and the warmed milk mixture and gently stir until the mixture thickens, 2 to 4 minutes. Remove from the heat and stir in the Cheddar, Gruyère, salt, and pepper. Add the cooked macaroni and stir to combine. Fold in the chopped tomatoes.

Mix the remaining 1 teaspoon oil with the breadcrumbs in a small bowl. Fill each muffin cup about three-fourths full with the pasta mixture and sprinkle each muffin with breadcrumbs.

Bake until the sauce bubbles and the macaroni has browned, 30 to 35 minutes. Cool for 5 minutes. Serve garnished with the thyme.

Nutrition facts per 2-muffin serving: 145 calories, 10 grams protein, 12 grams carbohydrates, 6 grams fat

Purple and Sweet Potato Fries

SERVES 8

Sweet potato fries are one of my new addictions and they taste amazing with my yogurt dip. If you can't find purple potatoes, just double the amount of sweet potatoes.

FRIES

1 pound purple potatoes (6 small)

1 pound sweet potatoes (3 medium)

1 tablespoon herbes de Provence

½ teaspoon fine sea salt

½ teaspoon cracked black pepper

YOGURT DIP

1 cup 0% or 2% Greek yogurt

1 teaspoon garlic powder

1 teaspoon fine sea salt

1 teaspoon cracked black pepper

¼ teaspoon cayenne pepper

¼ bunch flat-leaf parsley, chopped

To make the fries: Position a rack in the top third of the oven and preheat to 400°F. Coat a baking sheet with cooking spray.

Scrub the potatoes and cut lengthwise into ½-inch slices. Stack the slices and cut lengthwise into ½-inch-wide fries. Place the fries on the baking sheet and coat with cooking spray. Sprinkle the potatoes with the herbes de Provence, salt, and pepper and lightly toss to distribute the seasonings. Bake for 25 minutes, then flip with a spatula and coat again with cooking spray. Bake until golden brown, about 25 minutes. Cool for 5 minutes on the baking sheet.

Meanwhile, to make the dip: Stir together the yogurt, garlic powder, salt, black pepper, and cayenne in a medium bowl. Garnish with the parsley and serve with potato fries.

Nutrition facts per serving (1 cup fries and 2 tablespoons dip): 120 calories, 5 grams protein, 23 grams carbohydrates, 1 gram fat

PFC Hint: Enjoy with a lean protein such as a turkey burger. (I have a great turkey burger recipe in my book Skinny Chicks Don't Eat Salads.*)*

Espresso Martini

SERVES 1

Martini for dessert? Yes, please. I'll take this any day over a traditional chocolate martini, which has 2 shots of chocolate liqueur, 1 shot of vodka, and 4 ounces of heavy cream. That's 438 calories, 9 grams of fat, 42 grams of carbohydrates, and 28.5 grams sugar! Additional food for thought: One shot equals 1 ounce, so when you are preparing this drink use a shot glass instead of a measuring cup to keep it simple.

3 shots (1 ounce each) light coconut milk, plus extra for the rim

2 shots (1 ounce each) espresso or strong coffee

1 shot (1 ounce) vanilla vodka

1 shot (1 ounce) crème de cacao

10 dark chocolate-covered espresso beans, finely crushed

Dark chocolate shavings

Combine the coconut milk, espresso, vodka, and crème de cacao in a cocktail shaker with ice and shake until frothy. Put the extra coconut milk in a shallow dish, wider than the rim of the martini glass. Put the espresso beans in a separate dish. Dip the rim of the glass in the coconut milk and then in the ground beans. Fill with the shaken cocktail and sprinkle with dark chocolate shavings.

Nutrition facts per serving: 210 calories, 0 grams protein, 16 grams carbohydrates, 5 grams fat (all good fat!)

PFC Hint: Indulge after or with a PP meal or omit the carb from a PC meal.

Mojito Flaquito (a.k.a. Skinny Mojito)

SERVES 1

A perfect cocktail for summer! The recipe makes about ½ cup of simple syrup, much more than you need for one cocktail, but note that it will keep for weeks in a sealed container in the refrigerator.

½ cup coconut palm sugar

2 lime wedges

1 strawberry

A large handful of fresh mint sprigs

1½ ounces white rum

3½ ounces sparkling mineral water

Combine the sugar and ½ cup water in a medium saucepan. Bring to a boil and cook until the sugar is dissolved. Set the simple syrup aside to cool completely. (The simple syrup can be made up to 1 week ahead of time and stored in a covered container in the refrigerator.)

Combine 1 teaspoon simple syrup, 1 lime wedge, the strawberry and most of the mint sprigs in a tall glass. Use the handle of a wooden spoon or a muddler to crush the ingredients together, releasing their juices and oils. Add ice and top with the rum and sparkling water. Garnish with a lime wedge and fresh mint leaves.

Nutrition facts per serving: 86 calories, 0 grams protein, 8 grams carbohydrates, 0 grams fat

PFC Hint: Indulge after or with a PP meal or omit the carb from a PC meal.

Pomelo Martini

SERVES 1

Pomelo is a Chinese grapefruit with a really thick skin. Pomelos to me are the perfect compromise between an orange and a grapefruit. They are not as sweet as oranges yet they are not as tart as grapefruits. . . . They are absolutely lovely and it is fun to be a bit exotic with your food once in a while. If you cannot find it, please substitute regular grapefruit.

½ pomelo or grapefruit

1 shot (1 ounce) Grand Marnier or other orange-flavored liqueur

1 cup sparkling mineral water

Fresh mint leaf

With a vegetable peeler, pull off a strip of pomelo zest to use for garnish. Juice the pomelo to get ½ cup juice. Stir together the pomelo juice and Grand Marnier in a tall glass. Add ice and top off with the sparkling water. Garnish with a fresh mint leaf and the twist of pomelo zest.

Nutrition facts per serving: 150 calories, 1 gram protein, 18 grams carbohydrates, 0 grams fat

PFC Hint: Indulge after a PP meal or omit the carb from a PC meal.

Skinny Pomegranate Bellinis

SERVES 16

A delightful addition to a healthy Sunday brunch. Cheers!

2 cups Grand Marnier or other orange-flavored liqueur

1 cup pure pomegranate juice

1 bottle (750 ml) champagne or prosecco

8 thin orange slices, halved

½ cup pomegranate seeds

Pour the Grand Marnier and pomegranate juice into a large glass pitcher. Stir well and chill for 20 minutes.

For each bellini, pour about 3 tablespoons pomegranate mixture into a champagne flute and top with a scant ¼ cup of champagne or prosecco. Garnish with a half orange slice and a few pomegranate seeds and serve immediately.

Nutrition facts per 3.5-ounce serving: 160 calories, 0 grams protein, 12 grams carbohydrates, 0 grams fat

PFC Hint: Indulge after a PP meal or omit the carb from a PC meal.

Christine's Detox Tea

SERVES 5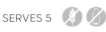

Artichoke extract is available at Amazon.com and helps with digestion and liver detoxification. Thirty drops is the equivalent of one dose.

3 ounces fresh ginger, peeled and sliced

3 dandelion root tea bags

3 milk thistle tea bags

2 cinnamon sticks

30 drops artichoke extract

2 tablespoons fresh lemon juice

Combine 5 cups of water and the ginger in a large saucepan. Bring to a gentle boil and boil for 1 minute. Remove from the heat. Add the tea bags and cinnamon sticks. Cover and steep for 15 minutes. Strain into a large pitcher. Add the artichoke extract and lemon juice. Stir and refrigerate for 30 minutes or until cold.

Nutrition facts per 1-cup serving: 4 calories, 0 grams protein, 1 gram carbohydrate, 0 grams fat

Free Drink: It's only 4 calories!

Recovery Veggie Shots

These shots are good for liver cell regeneration and increased bile flow. They also ease the headaches that can accompany detoxing, reduce free-radical damage, protect liver cells, and rid the body of toxins from the environment, drugs, and food additives. If you have a juicer you can simply juice all the ingredients together without roasting the beets or blanching the greens.

1 beet

1 cup dandelion greens (available at most farmers' markets)

1 cup broccoli florets

1 cup lightly packed spinach

¼ cup fresh cilantro

1 tomato, peeled (see Note) and seeded

¼ cup chopped scallions

1 cup Christine's Detox Tea (page 269)

Preheat the oven to 375°F. Wash the beet and wrap tightly in foil. Place on a foil-lined baking sheet and roast until tender enough to poke through easily with a knife, about 1 hour. When cool enough to handle, peel the beet and transfer to a blender.

While the beet roasts, bring a large pot of water to a boil. Strip the stems from the dandelion leaves. Add the broccoli to the boiling water and blanch for 4 minutes. Add the spinach and dandelion greens for the last 1 minute.

Add the blanched green veggies to the blender along with the cilantro, tomato, scallion, and tea and puree until very smooth. Strain the juice through a fine-mesh strainer into a glass pitcher. Serve immediately or chill for up to 1 hour before serving. Keep refrigerated for up to 2 days.

Nutrition facts per ¼-cup shot: 21 calories, 1 gram protein, 5 grams carbohydrates, 0 grams fat

Note: To peel the tomato, drop it into a pot of boiling water and boil for 1 minute. Rinse under cold water, then peel.

Free Drink: It's only 21 calories, but limit to 2 servings per day.

Acknowledgments

First I must thank Jesus Christ for blessing me with your grace, favor, abundance, and unconditional love—constantly giving me gifts that I don't deserve. Thank you for trusting me with this platform, I hope I can be a blessing and extension of your unconditional love for all people, all races, and all walks of faith.

Jonathon, my most special gift from heaven. Thank you for "seeing my heart" and teaching me what true love really is. You have been a huge part of this book . . . from making me laugh and smile at the cover shoot to patiently sitting with me at your office as I wrote until all hours of the night. You refused to leave my side . . . because that's just the way you are. Words cannot express how lucky I feel to have you in my life. You are my love, my best friend, and my inspiration.

An endless stream of thank you's and love to all of my clients in North America, Canada, South America, Germany, UK, Dubai, and Japan. I learn from you every day and without you I would have nothing to write about!

A very special heartfelt thank you to my agents at CAA, Christina Kuo, Stephanie Paciullo, who attended my first book signing only a few weeks after meeting me. From the start, you have been 110 percent on board with me professionally and personally. Simon Green, my literary agent, your support and advice is always spot on. My legal team Jeff Bernstein and Robert Koch, you guys are my super heroes, always guiding, guarding, and governing my opportunities, thank you so much for your extreme care and belief in me. All of you are beyond amazing and this book would have never been possible without your support. Thanks for standing by me through all the ups and downs . . . you are my family and I love all of you so very much.

A special thanks to Pam Krauss, the world's most gifted, coolest, and wonderful editor. Wow, Pam this has certainly been a journey for you and I, and I cannot thank you enough for always believing in me and my ideas. We have come a long way and I'm so glad you got on board with this real food diet concept from day one.

The amazing editing team at Rodale, Andrea Levitt, Zachary Greenwald, Victoria Glerum, and all the Rodale editors. You guys really kicked butt on this book, thanks for all of your hard work and attention to detail . . . I appreciate each of you so very much.

To my collaborating writer Bonnie Bauman, girl, from the moment we watched *Food Inc.* and had a good long cry, you have been on fire of this project, and I could not have found a better partner! Your amazing intellect in the subject of real food is mind-blowing. I'm so glad to have gone on this journey with you. You are a true superstar, and this book rocks because of your undying hard work.

To my culinary instructor, Chef Cecilia De Castro, thank you for teaching me "the basics" of classical French cooking. Not only did I graduate from your culinary program as a chef, but your teachings brought me back to my true love for REAL FOOD. You were a huge inspiration for this book.

My deepest gratitude to my friend and fellow chef Tiffany O'Reilly, thanks for all of your amazing work on the recipe development, editing, and for being a true friend in my darkest hours.

Daniese Jurado, Sheryl Bard, Kathrine England, and Steve Truitt, your teaching, counseling, prayers, support, and positive energy helped settle me and focus on this book—in the midst of a very challenging year—you are truly heaven sent!

Caroline Barnette, Merilee Kaszacs, Kallissa Miller, Linda Frost, Colet Abedi, Cathea Walters, Andrea Kelly, Joy Lindleif, and Amy Richenbach—thank you for standing by me and being amazing friends . . . your love and support have been a tremendous blessing to me . . . I love you ladies. It is rare to have friends who never judge and always encourage . . . thank you.

Cecilia Gutierrez (aka Nanny C), for researching, helping me rename all the recipes, researching, and helping with the real food grocery lists, taking special care of my baby boy Luigi, loving me, believing in me.

A big thank you to the Real Foodies who were gracious enough to contribute their real food knowledge for this book—Nina Plank, Mark Bittman, Lisa Leake, Kath Younger, Vin Miller, Sunshine Boatright, and Kristen Michaelis.

The folks at ITV—Joe Livecchi, Kenny Hull, Val Idehen, Doc, Alex Del Real, Jay Sinrod, Brett Hoebel, Robert Brace, and Dan Rafeld— thanks for being so fun to work with and supporting me on every level!! You guys are the bestest!!

To the nutritionistas who busted their butts on research, Robin Olsson, Cara Clark, and Sheila Campbell, thanks for your undying commitment to helping me with my research. Sheila, you stayed up with me 48 hours without sleeping several times to meet deadlines . . . I cannot find the words to express my gratitude.

To the gals who make me look so good. Joan Allen, you are the world's most awesome photographer, thanks for your creativity and genuine thoughtfulness with the book covers. I love you, Joanie! Shannon Wilson, my hair stylist, thank you for your amazing work over the years and for making my hair look so great on this cover. Vivianna Martin, the best makeup artist in the world—thank you for your love and prayers. Jasmine Robles of Byron and Tracy Salon in Beverly Hills, you are truly heaven sent—thank you for fresh, gorgeous blowout, you are amazing!

A loving thanks to my mom, Chris-Dad, Janine, Steve, Lily Zukowski, and Chris Green; you are my biggest heroes, supporters, listeners, and fans. I can't imagine this life without your endless love.

To all my families who have always cheered me on: the Avanti's, the Chiminello's, the Seaton's, the Surface's, the Fischers (Marina and Bob- thanks for your brainstorming on the subtitle!). A big hug to my wonderful Aunts: Mary, Louise, Gerry and Sandra-thanks for loving me and encouraging me for as long as I can remember.

Finally, Luigi, my only child. To the world you are a Labrador retriever, but to me you are my baby boy. Thank you for staying awake night after night with me as I wrote this book. You rescued me and healed my heart. I love you, Bubba.

APPENDIX A

A Feast of Real-Food Resources

Books

Learn More about Fat

Eat Fat Lose Fat, Mary Enig
Know Your Fats: The Complete Primer for Understanding the Nutrition of Fats, Oils and Cholesterol, Mary G. Enig
The Cholesterol Myths: Exposing the Fallacy That Saturated Fat and Cholesterol Cause Heart Disease, Uffe Ravnskov, MD

Learn More about Sugar

Skinny Chicks Don't Eat Salads, Christine Avanti
Ending the Food Fight, Dr. David Ludwig
Good Calories, Bad Calories, Gary Taubes

Real Food in the Kitchen

Nourishing Traditions, Sally Fallon & Mary Enig
In the Green Kitchen, Alice Waters
Complete Book of Home Preserving, edited by Judi Kingry and Lauren Devine
The Food Matters Cookbook, Mark Bittman

My Go-to Real-Food Gurus

What to Eat, Marion Nestle
Food Matters, Mark Bittman
The Omnivore's Dilemma, Michael Pollan
Food Rules, Michael Pollan
In Defense of Food, Michael Pollan
Real Food: What to Eat and Why, Nina Planck
Real Food for Mother and Baby, Nina Planck

My Favorite Wellness Warriors

Staying Well in a Toxic World, Lynn Lawson
You on a Diet, Dr. Michael Roizen, Dr. Mehmet Oz
The End of Overeating, Dr. David Kessler

Blog Roll

www.foodpolitics.com
www.100daysofrealfood.com
www.naturalbias.com
www.katheats.com/kathrd
www.realfoodrehab.blogspot.com
www.lifeasaplate.com
www.101cookbooks.com

www.realfoodhascurves.com
www.eatingrealfood.com
www.realfoodrenegade.com
www.nourishedkitchen.com
www.unitedstatesoffood.com
www.simplysugarandglutenfree.com
www.realfoodlover.wordpress.com
www.realfoodwholehealth.com
www.injennieskitchen.com
www.markbittman.com
www.keepingitrealfood.com
www.brooklynhomesteader.com
www.nourishingdays.com
www.thehealthyhomeeconomist.com

Documentaries

Food, Inc.
The Future of Food
Super Size Me

APPENDIX B

Real Food on a Budget

Depending on where you live, you might not have access to Whole Foods Market, a farmers' market, or other natural food stores. With this in mind, I created a shopping list of real foods available at Walmart, Costco, and Trader Joe's. Please note that these items are not the only real foods available at these stores. Also, product availability will vary from location to location. It is most certainly possible that you will find other wonderful real foods that are not on this list. This list is just a guide to get you into the store with confidence as you embark upon your real-food diet journey. I hope you find it helpful.

Real Foods at Walmart

FREEZER CASE

Frozen Fruits: Dole Ready-Cut Fruit, Wildly Nutritious Mixed Berries, 100% Pineapple Chunks; Great Value Berry Medley, Whole Strawberries, Blueberries, Red Raspberries, Blackberries, Crushed Pineapple; Nature's Peak Wild Blueberries; Sunrise Growers Dark Sweet Cherries

Frozen Vegetables: Bird's Eye Steamfresh Frozen Vegetables, Baby Potato Blend, Broccoli, Sweet Peas, Green Beans, Brussels Sprouts, Corn; C&W Pepper Strips, Chopped Spinach, Zucchini; Great Value Steamable Peas, Broccoli and Cauliflower, Broccoli Cuts, Mixed Vegetables, Crinkle Cut Carrots, Deluxe Stir Fry; Green Giant Valley Fresh Steamers, Broccoli Florets, Whole Green Beans, Cut Green Beans, White Shoepeg Corn, Sugar Snap Peas, Cut Green Beans; Pictsweet Chopped Green Peppers, Whole Okra, Broccoli, Brussels Sprouts, Collard Greens, Turnip Greens

GRAINS, CEREALS, LEGUMES, BREADS, AND CRACKERS AISLE

Cereals: Great Value 100% Natural Whole Grain Old Fashioned Oats; John McCanns' Steel Cut Irish Oatmeal; Quaker Oats Natural Whole Grain Rolled Oats

Grains and Rice: Great Value Whole Grain Brown Rice; Wild Roots 100% Milled Golden Flaxseeds; Annie Chun's Rice Noodles

CANNED GOODS AISLE

Canned Vegetables: Great Value Collard Greens, Turnip Greens, Corn

SWEETENERS

Agave nectar; honey

CONDIMENTS AND SAUCES

Various vinegars; HFCS-free ketchup; pasta sauces (read labels, must have all real food and pronounceable ingredients); low-sodium, MSG-free soy sauce

OILS

Lou Ann Pure Coconut Oil; extra-virgin olive oil (various brands); sesame oil

NUTS

Blue Diamonds Whole Natural Almonds; Chef's Naturals Slivered Almonds Dry Roasted, Macadamias, Almonds, Pine Nuts, Natural Sliced Almonds; Diamond Sliced Almonds; Emerald 100 Calorie Packs Natural Almonds; Fisher Pecan Chips

DRIED FRUITS

Wild Roots Mango Slices, Mixed Berries

BEVERAGES

Lipton Tea Bags; various coffee brands

Real Foods at Costco
(Yes, You Can Buy Real Food in Bulk!)

REFRIGERATOR CASE

Fresh Meats: Coastal Range Organics Ground Turkey, Chicken Breasts, Wild Caught Alaskan Salmon, a variety of other wild caught seafood

Dairy: Kirkland Organic Salted Butter; Fage Total 100% All Natural Non-Fat Greek Style Yogurt

FREEZER CASE

Grains: Rice Expressions Rice Express Natural Brown Rice

Frozen Fruits: Kirkland Signature Rader Farms Nature's Three Berries, Strawberries; Townsend Farms Dark Sweet Cherries and Organic Blackberries; Wawona Frozen Foods Festival Blend

Frozen Fish: Kirkland Signature Wild Caught Sockeye Salmon, Wild Alaska Pacific Cod and Tilapia Loins, Wild Pacific Mahi-Mahi; Seamazz North Atlantic Lobster Tails

Frozen Vegetables: Bybee Foods Organic Mixed Vegetables; Kirkland Signature Stir-Fry Vegetable Blend, Normandy Style Vegetable Blend; Madame Edamame 100% Natural Soybeans, Pure Nature Broccoli Florets

GRAINS, LEGUMES, BREADS, AND CRACKERS AISLE

Cereals: Coach's Oats 100% Whole Grain Oatmeal; Nature's Path Organic Ancient Grains, Granola with Almonds, Organic Pumpkin Flax Plus Granola; Quaker Oats Old Fashioned

Dry Goods: Alpine Valley Organic Whole Grain Bread

Rice: Cooked brown rice bowls

CANNED GOODS AISLE

Canned Meats: Bear and Wolf Wild Alaskan Salmon; Chicken of the Sea Chunk Light Tuna in Water; Kirkland Alaskan Sockeye Salmon, Season Sardines in Pure Olive Oil; Tonno Solid Light Tuna in Olive Oil

Canned Vegetables: Kirkland Golden Sweet Corn, Fancy Grade Green Beans

Other: Tree Toppers Apple Sauce (with absorbic acid, a.k.a. vitamin C)

SWEETENERS
Busy Bee Pure Organic Honey; Kirkland Grade A Medium Amber Maple Syrup; Wholesome Sweeteners Organic Blue Agave

CONDIMENTS AND SAUCES
Mario Batali Pasta Sauce; Kirkland Organic Salsa, balsamic vinegar, red wine vinegar

OILS
Extra-virgin olive oil

NUTS
Nuts: Hoody's Roasted In-Shell Peanuts; Kirkland Signature Pine Nuts, Almonds, Walnuts, Pecans, Dry Roasted Almonds; Planters Dry Roasted Peanuts

Nut Butters: Mara Natha All Natural Roasted Almond Butter; Kirkland Organic Creamy Peanut Butter

DRIED FRUITS
Sun Dates California Medjool Dates; Hadley Pitted Deglet Noor Dates

BEVERAGES
Various dried teas and organic coffees; Bolthouse Farms Carrot Juice; Sanbazon Acai; Vita Coco 100% Pure Coconut Water with Vitamin C

Trader Joe's (My Personal Fave!)

REFRIGERATOR CASE
Dairy: Kerrgold Irish Butter, Cabot Cheddar; Trader Joe's Organic Milk; Organic Whole Milk Mozzarella, Organic Sheep's Milk Feta, Grated Parmigiano-Reggiano (made with raw milk and animal rennet), Cottage Cheese, Ciliegine Whole Milk Fresh Mozzarella (I live on this stuff!); Raita Indian Style Yogurt; Red Carton Organic Full Fat Yogurt; Fage Greek Non-Fat and 1% Greek Yogurt

Eggs: Trader Joe's Organic Free-Range Eggs and Fertile Eggs (Cage Free)

Meats and Fish: Trader Joe's Apple Wood Smoked Uncured Thick Sliced Bacon, Chili Lime Chicken Burgers, Organic Free-Range Chicken, Uncooked American Style Kobe Beef Burgers (Wagyu Beef), 100% Grass Fed Ground Beef, Wild-Caught Salmon and Tilapia (neither on endangered list), Buffalo Burgers; Atkins Ranch New Zealand Lamb Grass Fed

Vegetable Preparations: Asian Stir-Fry Healthy 9 Chopped Veggie Mix, Julienned Sautéed Steamed Lentils and Steamed Baby Beets, Organic Arugula, Organic Baby Spinach, and many other organic and local produce options!

Spreads: Trader Joe's Organic Hummus and Organic Garlic Hummus

FREEZER CASE

Frozen Fruit: Organic Berry Medley, Organic Raspberry Medley, Organic Wild Blueberries, Pineapple Tidbits and Raspberries

Frozen Vegetables: Trader Joe's Broccoli Florets, Carrots Rustica (yellow and orange carrots), Chopped Spinach, Fire Roasted Bell Peppers and Onions, Grilled Asparagus Spears, Melange a Trois (red, yellow, and green bell pepper strips), Petite Peas, Organic Green Beans, Haricots Verts (extra-fine French green beans), Organic Foursome (sweet white corn, sweet peas, julienned carrots and green beans), Organic Super Sweet Corn and Roasted Corn

Grains: Trader Joe's Brown Rice Bags (frozen)

Frozen Meals: Trader Joe's Indian Fare Polak Paneer, Pav Bhaji and Punjab Choley, Shrimp Stir-Fry and Tuna in Red Panang Curry Sauce

GRAINS, LEGUMES, BREADS, AND CRACKERS AISLE

Pasta: Trader Joe's Organic Brown Rice Spaghetti, Whole Wheat Spaghetti, Penne, Rotelle and Wheat Durum Pasta

Cereal and Grains: Bob's Red Mill Whole Ground Flaxseed Meal; Lindberg Organic Brown Rice Cakes; McCann's Steel Cut Oatmeal and Quick Cooking Rolled Irish Oatmeal; Trader Joe's Quick Cook Steel Cut Oats; Natural Toasted Oat Bran, Organic Pumpkin Flax Plus Granola, Shredded Bite Size Wheat

Breads, Crackers, and Tortillas: Ak-mak 100% Organically Grown Whole Wheat Flour Sesame Crackers; Ezekiel 4:9 100% Whole Grain

Bread and Low-Sodium Sesame Cinnamon Raisin Bread; Food for Life Brown Rice Bread; Trader Joe's Rye, No Flour Sprout Wheat Berry, Sprouted Barley, Organic Flourless, Sprouted 7-Grain Bread, Sprouted Multi-Grain, Harvest Whole Wheat Bread, 100% Whole Grain Fiber Whole Wheat, Whole Wheat Honey Bread, European Style Whole Grain Bread, French Village Plus 100% Stone Ground Whole Grain Bread, Whole Wheat Pita Bread, Sheppard's Bread, Clay Oven Baked Whole Wheat Lavash Bread

Tortillas: Trader Joe's Blue Corn Tortillas Organic and Corn Tortillas Made from Freshly Ground Corn

CANNED GOODS AISLE

Soups: Trader Joe's Organic Hearty Vegetable Broth, Split Pea Soup, True Thai Tom Yam Soup

Jarred Fruits: Trader Joe's First Crush Unsweetened Gravenstein Apple Sauce, Chunk Spice Apples

Canned Vegetables: Trader Joe's Organic Canned Cut Green Beans, Garbanzo Beans, Pinto Beans, Refried Beans, Whole Kernel Corn

SWEETENERS

Stevia, honey, maple syrup

CONDIMENTS AND SAUCES

Pasta Sauce: Trader Giotto's Puttanesca Sauce Made With Italian Tomatoes and Organic Marinara, Organic Tomato Basil Marinara, Recipe #99 Traditional Marinara Sauce, Organic Vodka Sauce, Roasted Organic Spaghetti Sauce, and Trader Joe's Marinara Sauce

Salsas: Trader Joe's Hot Chipotle Salsa, Organic Tomatillo Roasted Yellow Chili Salsa, Smokey Peach Salsa, Salsa Authentica, Salsa Verde

Basic Condiments: Trader Joe's Organic Ketchup, Real Mayonnaise

OILS

Extra-virgin olive oil; olive oil spray; sesame oil

NUTS

All Trader Joe's raw nuts including almonds, dry-roasted almonds, organic almonds, unsalted slivered almonds, sliced almonds, salted skin-on Marcona almonds, Brazil nuts, raw whole cashews, roasted unsalted cashews, organic dry-roasted and lightly salted cashews, dry-roasted and salted pistachios, pumpkin seeds in-shell, salted pepitas, raw sunflower seeds, California Walnut Baking Pieces, raw walnut halves and pieces

Nut Butters: Trader Joe's Almond Butter Raw Creamy, Almond Butter with Sea Salt, Unsalted and Crunch Unsalted Peanut Butter from Unbleached Peanuts, Trader Joe's Almond Butter Raw Crunchy Unsalted

DRIED FRUITS

Trader Joe's Freeze Dried Fruits: Strawberries, Blueberries; Trader Joe's Nothing But Banana Flattened, Organic Thompson Seedless Raisins, Just Mango Slices, New Zealand Sweet Apple Rings, Turkish Smyrna Figs (unsulfured)

Fruit Bars: All Fruit Bars Handmade 100% Dried Fruit Bars and Pieces Assorted Flavors; Greens+ Chocolate Energy Bar, Pure Organic Cherry Cashew Bar; Lärabars Apple Pie, Cashew Cookie, Chocolate Brownie Bar, Peanut Butter, Cherry Pie, Peanut Butter Chocolate Chip

BEVERAGES

Various dried teas, organic coffees, and herbal teas; Trader Joe's Organic Unsweetened Soy Milk; Westsoy Organic Unsweetened Soy Milk; Trader Joe's Light Coconut Milk

References

Chapter 1

Colantuoni, C., J. Schwenker, P. McCarthy, et al. 2001. "Excessive Sugar Intake Alters Binding to Dopamine and μ-Opioid Receptors in the Brain." *NeuroReport* 12(16): 3549–52.

Harding, Matthew. 2010. "Junk Food's Addictiveness Re-evaluated." *DigitalJournal.com*, March 29. http://digitaljournal.com/article/289768.

Harmon, Katherine. 2010. "Addicted to Fat: Overeating May Alter the Brain as Much as Hard Drugs." *Scientific American Online*, March 28. http://www.scientificamerican.com/article.cfm?id=addicted-to-fat-eating.

Kessler, Gary. 2009. *The End of Overeating*. New York: Rodale.

Moeller, Rachael. 2011. "Addicted to Food?" *Eating Well*, March/April.

Johnson, P., and P.J. Kenny. 2010. "Dopamine D2 Receptors in Addiction-like Reward Dysfunction and Compulsive Eating in Obese Rats." *Nature Neuroscience* 13(5): 635–41.

Vucetic, Z., J. Kimmel, T.M. Reyes. 2011. "Chronic High-fat Diet Drives Postnatal Epigenetic Regulation of μ-Opioid Receptor in the Brain." *Neuropsychopharmacology* 36(6): 1199–1206.

Chapter 2

Kimbrell, Andrew, ed. 2002. *Fatal Harvest: The Tragedy of Industrial Agriculture*. Sausolito, CA: Foundation for Deep Ecology by arrangement with Island Press.

Levenstein, Harvey. 2003. *Paradox of Plenty: A Social History of Eating in Modern America*. Berkeley: University of California Press.

Morell, Sally Fallon. 2011. "Dirty Secrets of the Food Processing Industry." *Well Being Journal*, March/April.

Nestle, Marion. 2006. *What to Eat*. New York: North Point Press.

Pollan, Michael. 2008. *In Defense of Food*. New York: Penguin.

Pollan, Michael. 2001. *The Omnivore's Dilemma*. New York: Penguin.

Schlosser, E. 2001. Fast Food Nation: The Dark Side of the All-American Meal. New York: Houghton Mifflin.

Smith, Jeffrey M. 2003. *Seeds of Deception*. New York: Yes Books.

Whitman, Deborah B. 2000. "Genetically Modified Foods: Harmful or Helpful?" *CSA Discovery Guides*, April.

Chapter 3

Avanti, Christine. 2009. *Skinny Chicks Don't Eat Salads*. New York: Rodale.

Kleinfield, N.R. 2006. "Diabetes and Its Awful Toll Quietly Emerge as a Crisis." *New York Times*, January 9.

Ludwig, David. 2008. *Ending the Food Fight*. New York: Mariner Books.

Nestle, Marion. 2006. *What to Eat*. New York: North Point Press.

Price, Weston A. 2008. *Nutrition and Physical Regeneration*. New York: Price Pottenger Nutrition.

Taubes, Gary. 2007. *Good Calories, Bad Calories*. New York: Knopf.

Chapter 4

Cordain, Loren. 2010. *The Paleo Diet*. New York: Wiley.

Enig, Mary G., and Sally Fallon. 2006. *Eat Fat, Lose Fat*. New York: Plume.

Kendrick, Malcolm. 2008. *The Great Cholesterol Con*. New York: John Blake.

Planck, Nina. 2007. *Real Food: What to Eat and Why*. New York: Bloomsbury.

Price, Weston A. 2008. *Nutrition and Physical Regeneration*. New York: Price Pottenger Nutrition.

Ravnskov, Uffe. 2000. *The Cholesterol Myths*. New York: Newtrends Publishing Inc.

Chapter 6

Avanti, Christine. 2009. *Skinny Chicks Don't Eat Salads*. New York: Rodale.

Fallon, Sally, and Mary Enig. 2007. *Nourishing Traditions*. Washington, DC: New Trends Publishing.

Hansen, Evie. 2007. *Seafood: Omega-3s for Healthy Living*. Richmond Beach, Washington: National Seafood Educators.

Taubes, Gary. 2007. *Good Calories, Bad Calories*. New York: Knopf.

Chapter 7

Ebbeling, Cara B., Kelly B. Sinclair, Mark A. Pereira, Erica Garcia-Lago, Henry A. Feldman, David S. Ludwig. 2004. "Compensation for Energy Intake

From Fast Food Among Overweight and Lean Adolescents." *The Journal of the American Medical Association* 291(23): 2828–33.

Kessler, Gary. 2009. *The End of Overeating*. New York: Rodale.

Lally, Phillippa, Cornelia H.M. van Jaarsveld, Henry W. Potts, and Jane Wardle. 2010. "How Are Habits Formed: Modelling Habit Formation in the Real World." *European Journal of Social Psychology* 40(6): 998–1009.

Avena, Nicole M., Pedro Rada, Bartley G. Hoebel. 2008. "Review Evidence for Sugar Addiction: Behavioral and Neurochemical Effects of Intermittent, Excessive Sugar Intake." *Neuroscience and Biobehavioral Reviews* (Princeton University) 32:20–39.

Quinn, J.M., A. Pascoe, W. Wood, and D.T. Neal. 2010. "Can't Control Yourself? Monitor Those Bad Habits." *Perspectives in Social Psychology Bulletin* 36(4): 499–511.

Rothman, Alexander J., Paschal Sheeran, and Wendy Wood. 2009. "Reflective and Automatic Processes in the Initiation and Maintenance of Dietary Change," *Annals of Behavioral Medicine* 38: Suppl. no. 1, 4–17.

Chapter 8

Planck, Nina. 2007. *Real Food: What to Eat and Why*. New York: Bloomsbury.

Silverglade, Bruce, and Ilene Heller. 2010. *Food Labeling Chaos*. Washington, DC: Center for Science in the Public Interest.

Taubes, Gary. 2007. *Good Calories, Bad Calories*. New York: Knopf.

Chapter 9

Bittman, Mark. 2009. *Food Matters: A Guide to Conscious Eating*. New York: Simon & Schuster.

Bittman, Mark. 2008. "A Seafood Snob Ponders the Future of Fish." *New York Times*, November 15.

Bittman, Mark. 2009. "Loving Fish, This Time with the Fish in Mind." *New York Times*, June 9.

Blonz, Ed. 2009. "Skim Milk: Not a Health Hazard." *Daily Herald* (Chicago), February 4, 2009.

The Cornucopia Institute. 2009. *Behind the Barn: The Heroes and Charlatans of the Natural and Organic Soy Foods Industry*. Cornucopia, WI: The

Cornucopia Institute. www.cornucopia.org/2009/05/soy-report-and -scorecard/.

Anderson-Gips, Rose, comp. 2008. "Decoding Food Labels." Earthwatch Institute. www.earthwatch2.org/sustainability/decodinglabels.htm.

Johnson, Rachel K., and Lawrence J. Appel, et al. 2009. "Dietary Sugars Intake and Cardiovascular Health: A Scientific Statement from the American Heart Association." *Circulation* 120(11): 1011–20.

United States Department of Agriculture Food Safety and Inspection Service. 2006. "Meat and Poultry Labeling Terms." United States Department of Agriculture. www.fsis.usda.gov.factsheets/Meat_& _Poultry_Labeling_Terms/index.asp.

Monterey Bay Aquarium Seafood Watch 1999–2011, Monterey Bay Aquarium Foundation, 886 Cannery Row, Monterey, California. www.montereybayaquarium.org.

Nestle, Marion. 2010. "Bisphenol A (BPA): The Fuss Goes On and On." *FoodPolitics.com*, October 1. www.foodpolitics.com/2010/10 /bisphenol-a-bpa-the-fuss-goes-on-and-on/.

Nestle, Marion. 2006. *What to Eat.* New York: North Point Press.

Nestle, Marion. 2011. "Surprise! Most 'Better-for-You' Kids' Foods Aren't." *FoodPolitics.com*, January 19. www.foodpolitics.com/2011/01 /surprise-most-better-for-you-kids-food-arent/.

Pollan, Michael. 2008. *In Defense of Food.* New York: Penguin.

Pollan, Michael. 2006. *The Omnivore's Dilemma.* New York: Penguin.

Silverglade, Bruce, and Ilene Heller. 2010. *Food Labeling Chaos.* Washington, DC: Center for Science in the Public Interest.

The Whole Grains Council, Oldways, 266 Beacon Street, Boston, Massachusetts. http://www.wholegrainscouncil.org.

Waters, A.E., and T. Contente-Cuomo, et al. 2011. "Multidrug-Resistant *Staphylococcus aureus* in US Meat and Poultry." *Clinical Infectious Diseases* 52(10): 1227–30.

University of Arkansas Division of Agriculture Cooperative Extension Service. 2008. "What Does "Certified Organic" Really Mean?" University of Arkansas Division of Agriculture.

Chapter 10

Paska, Megan. 2011. "Food Swaps as Culinary Incubators and Food Factories." *Huffington Post*, March 28.

Appendix B

www.eartheasy.com

INDEX

Underscored page references indicate boxed text. An asterisk (*) indicates that photos are shown in the insert pages.

F

Factory food
  fats in (see industrial fats)
  health effects, 4–7
  history of, 14–15
  organic ingredients in, 120
  real food substitutions, 108
  salt in, 6–7, 66–67
  sugar in, 29, 64–66
Farming practices
  animal husbandry, 17–18, 42,
    124–25, 126, 128–29, 134
  biodynamic, 127
  traditional vs. monocultural, 16–17
Fast food, 98, 101
Fat Blaster Weight Loss Plan, 177–84
Fat-melting foods, 167, 171
Fats, in real foods. See also Industrial
    fats
  chemical composition, 41
  combining with protein/carbs,
    61–62, 160–61, 166
  cooking with, 45
  health benefits, 40
  label information, 38, 115–16, 118
  negative reputation, 39–40
  nutritional role, 38, 43
  portion sizes, 160, 165–66
  recommended types, 42, 144
Fat-soluble vitamins, 38
Fatty acids. See Essential fatty acids
FDA. See Food and Drug
    Administration (FDA)
Fennel, 151, 162
Fermented foods
  daily recommendations, 173, 178
  health benefits, 167, 170–71
Fiber
  label information, 110
  sources of, 69, 162–63
  synthetic, 108, 110
  water-soluble/insoluble, 69–71
  weight loss role, 68–72
Fish and seafood
  Chef Cece's Bouillabaisse, 234
  Cilantro-Lime Shrimp with Spicy
    Rice Noodles,* 244–45

Easy Lobster Pasta,* 243
  Greek Isles Salad, 224
  Grilled Halibut with Tomato
    Coulis,* 232
  Grilled Salmon, 179
  oils from, 42
  omega-3 source, 73, 163–64
  Quick Tuna Sandwich, 181
  Roasted Salmon, 183
  shopping guides, 128–31
  Spicy Tuna Poke, 219
  Zesty Citrus Halibut, 233
Flaxseeds/flaxseed oil, 42, 163
"Flipping your script," 85–86
Flour
  gluten free, 249
  wheat, 20–21, 111–12
Food addiction
  biological aspects, 4–6, 80–81
  emotional aspects, 9, 88–90
  overview, 8–10
  rehab tools
    awareness, 81–83
    competing behaviors, 83–85
    competing thoughts, 85–86
    overview, 79–80, 90
    support systems, 87
Food and Drug Administration
    (FDA), 98, 109–11, 136
Food-borne illnesses, 136
Food diaries, 10, 81–83, 91–98
Food preparation tips, 143, 168–69
"Frankenfoods," 17
Free radicals, 41
"Free range" labels, 120–21, 126
Frozen food, 141, 156, 168
Fructose, 29
Fruit. See also specific fruits
  Açaí Superfood Smoothie, 207
  Bangin' Banana Bread,* 201
  Christine's Fave Coconut
    Smoothie, 180, 208
  Cocoberry Cupcakes,* 250–51
  Coconut Espresso Smoothie, 182
  Coconut "Faux"gurt, 205
  as complex carbohydrate, 62
  dried, 70, 114

polyunsaturated oils, 42, 46, 96
processing effects, 46
trans fats, 47, 49, 67, 111
Insulin, 27. *See also* Blood sugar
levels
Insulin-like growth factor (IGF-1), 135
Inulin, 171
Isolated fibers, 110

J
Journaling, 10, 90. *See also* Food
diaries
Juices
orange juice, 20
Recovery Veggie Shots, 270

K
Kale
Hunger Buster food, 185
nutritional role, 131, 164
Kefir, 62, 204
Keys, Ancel, 39
Kidney function, 72
Kids, real food diet and, 191
Kiwi, nutritional role, 70, 132, 151
Kohlrabi, 185

L
Label information
diet food statements, 115–17
for meat/poultry, 123–28
misleading statements, 109–11
nutrition facts, 117–20
organic/natural statements,
120–23
overview, 108–9
for seafood, 129–30
for whole grains, 110, 111–14
Lamb
Grilled Lamb Chops, 181
Herb-Crusted Rack of Lamb with
Açaí Sauce,* 240–41
Lard, 40, 42, 45
Lauric acid, 170, 205

LDL, 40, 49
Leake, Lisa, 13–14, 22–24
Lecithin, 102
Leeks, 132, 185
Legumes. *See* Beans and legumes
Lemons, 132
Lentils, 162
Lettuce
Hunger Buster food, 185
nutritional role, 132, 163
Linoleic/linolenic acid, 41
Lipid hypothesis, 39
Local Harvest, 153
"Local" labels, 127
Lunches
to-go recommendations, 167–68
meal plans, 97–98, 173–78,
178–83
Lysine, 19–20

M
Macadamia nut oil, 42
Macronutrients, balance of, 43,
61–62, 118, 160–61
Margarine, 39, 47, 115
Meal frequency, 63
Meal planning
four-hour eating interval, 161–62,
172
guidelines for, 74–75, 172–73, 178
preparation days, 76–77, 168–69
Real-Food Fat Blaster Plan,
177–84
Real-Food Weight Loss Diet,
173–77
Meats. *See also specific meats*
cured, 101, 125, 194, 196
grass fed/pasture raised, 18,
120–21, 125–27
label information, 121, 123–28
portion sizes, 165
shopping guides, 153
Mercury, in seafood, 129, 130
Metabolism
coconut oil and, 166–67, 169–70
of sugar, 171